Tower Hamlets College
Learning Centre

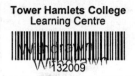

132009

Withdrawn

AN INTRODUCTORY GUIDE TO

Massage

THE LIBRARY
TOWER HAMLETS COLLEGE
POPLAR HIGH STREET
LONDON E14 0AF
Tel: 0207 510 7763

Louise Tucker

General Editor Jane Foulston

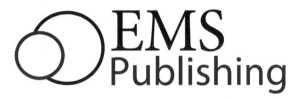
EMS
Publishing

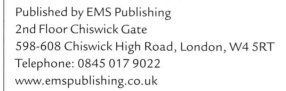

Published by EMS Publishing
2nd Floor Chiswick Gate
598-608 Chiswick High Road, London, W4 5RT
Telephone: 0845 017 9022
www.emspublishing.co.uk

© Education and Media Services Ltd.

The right of Louise Tucker to be identified as author of her
Work has been asserted by her in accordance with the Copyright,
Designs and Patents Act 1988.

All rights reserved; no part of this publication may be reproduced,
stored in a retrieval system, or transmitted in any form or by any
means, electronic, mechanical, photocopying, recording or
otherwise without the prior written permission of the Publishers.

First published November 2001
Second Edition October 2008
Revised January 2010
Third Edition July 2013

ISBN 978 1 903348 35 2

Printed by Bell & Bain Limited

Prepared for the publishers by Idego Media Limited.

Contents

Order No:
Class: 615.822 TUC
Accession No: 132009
Type: L

Introduction   v

Part one: Massage – from history to practical

1.   The history of massage and its use   7
2.   Anatomy for massage   11
3.   Massage techniques   29
4.   Effects and benefits of massage   73
5.   Professional conduct and consultation   81

Part two: Massage – uses and types

6.   Using on-site massage to treat stress   105
7.   What is Lymphatic drainage massage   115
8.   Infant and child massage   129
9.   Stone therapy massage   141
10. Indian head massage   177
11. Sports massage   193
12. Other complementary therapies   223

Bibliography   231
Glossary   232
Index   237

Acknowledgements

The publishers would like to thank the following people for their invaluable assistance in the preparation of this book:

Christine Clinton for Infant and Child Massage images
Brummell Associates
Isabella Panattoni Photographer
Jacqueline Jebb
Kay Galbraith for Indian Head and On-Site Massage routines
The Light Studios Studio space

And to the following models:
Karolina Palasinski
Michelle Dixon
Rachael Kammerling
Sheetal Bhatt

Introduction

An Introductory Guide to Massage is aimed at all those starting a career in the holistic therapy of massage. Covering all the required information for carrying out a treatment, including basic anatomy, techniques and benefits, it also provides an introduction to different types of massage, such as lymphatic drainage and Indian head. It is intended for use as a textbook, as part of an accredited course, and should not be considered a substitute for professional experience and qualifications.

Note for lecturers and students

This book has been produced primarily for use by students following the BTEC, City & Guilds, ITEC and VTCT massage syllabuses. As the publishers, we are aware, however, that there are a number of differing, and sometimes even conflicting, views on how the subject should be taught, the depth of subject matter which should be covered, and the manner in which it should be explained.

Whilst we welcome its use by anyone teaching massage therapy, we would urge lecturers and students alike to bear in mind that no textbook can be all things to all people. If, as a practising therapist or lecturer, you would like to submit comments on the book which may enable us to improve future editions, they will be warmly received. We regret, however, that we are unable to enter into a discussion with regard to the accuracy or appropriacy of our interpretation.

EMS Publishing

Author

Louise Tucker

Louise Tucker is a freelance writer and teacher. She has written and published several books and articles.

General editor

Jane Foulston

Jane Foulston has been in the beauty and complementary therapy industry for over 26 years. Jane taught beauty and complementary therapies in both further education and the private sector for 14 years. She then set up a beauty therapy college in Japan before working nationally and internationally as an ITEC examiner. Since becoming its Director in 1998, ITEC has gone on to become the world's largest international awarding body for beauty therapy.

Contributing editors

Elaine Hall

Elaine Hall began her career teaching beauty and complementary therapies at the West of England College in Bath. She then went on to manage the complementary therapies section at Bridgwater College. Since then Elaine has run her own private salon and clinic based within a nursing home. In addition she has held the post of senior ITEC examiner and she examines extensively both in the South West of England and overseas.

Fae Major

Fae Major has worked in the beauty therapy industry for 23 years. Her experience has included working for Steiner's and alternative medicine clinics, as well as private beauty salons in the UK and Barbados. Fae has 15 years teaching experience and became a practical examiner for ITEC in 1992. As well as continuing to examine, Fae is currently working for ITEC as part of the Qualifications Development team.

Lorinda Taylor

Lorinda Taylor has been an examiner for ITEC for the last 5 years, having worked in the industry for over 15. Qualified in Complementary and Beauty Therapies, Lorinda now runs her own practice. She has taught in a variety of educational settings for both the private and state education sectors and currently lectures for a group of colleges.

Jill Wilshaw

Jill Wilshaw qualified in Beauty Therapy in 1980. Initially she worked in a top London Slimming Clinic before opening up her own highly successful home visiting practice in and around Harrogate. During this time she started her own private school teaching mainly Anatomy, Physiology and Massage. After relocating to Aberdeen she lectured in many subjects relating to Beauty, Complementary and Sports Therapies at Aberdeen College. She has been a Senior Examiner for ITEC in both practical and theory since 1983.

Marguerite Wynne

Marguerite Wynne began her career in one of London's foremost beauty salons and went on to teach in the College of Beauty Therapy in London. Subsequently she owned her own salon and school in Buckinghamshire and at the same time worked as Chief Examiner for ITEC. In 2005 Marguerite was appointed Education Manager for ITEC where she now monitors the standards and consistency of ITEC examinations.

1 The history of massage and its use

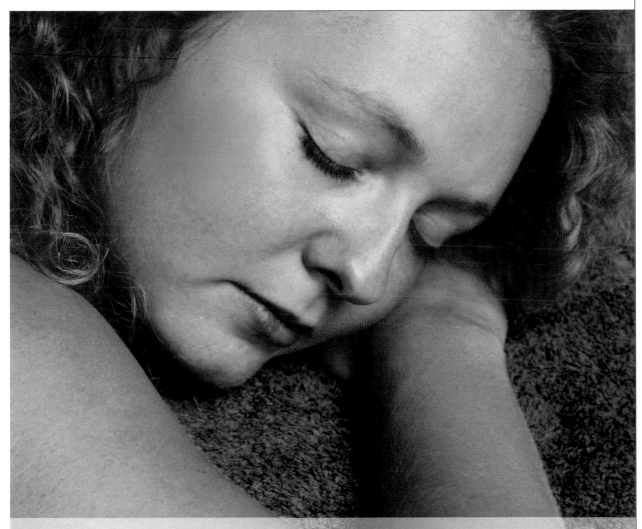

In Brief

Massage is a form of manipulation of the soft tissues of the body which has developed over thousands of years. From ancient China to present-day Europe it has been used for the promotion and restoration of health.

Learning objectives

The target knowledge of this chapter is:
● the history and origins of massage.

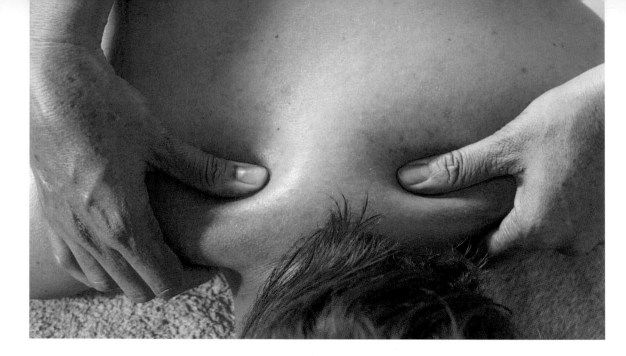

What is massage?

Massage is the use of hands, or mechanical means, to manipulate the soft tissues of the body, particularly muscles. It can be used for relaxation, stimulation or rehabilitation of the whole body or part of it. It promotes suppleness of the muscles, improves circulation and reduces stress.

What are its main benefits and effects?

Massage is:

- *soothing:* touch is known to be soothing and comforting and massage uses touch to soothe and relax the body. Since 75% of disease is thought to be caused by stress, massage, which reduces stress, may well improve health.
- *stimulating:* the systems of the body are stimulated and activated by massage. It therefore encourages improved circulation, aids digestion, waste removal and neural communication, invigorates and relaxes muscles thus preventing spasm and stiffness, speeds up skin desquamation and promotes cell regeneration.
- *instinctive:* when we knock or hurt ourselves we often use our hands to rub or touch the affected place. Massage is an extension of this natural and instinctive method of soothing aches and pains.
- *comforting:* touch is natural and comforting. People of all ages use touch to gain a sense of security and well-being and consequently massage has psychological as well as physiological benefits.
- *universal:* most people, from children to adults, can benefit from massage treatments.
- *safe:* massage is a non-threatening, non-invasive and natural therapy.

See Chapter 3 for more detailed information on the benefits and effects of massage.

Where does it come from?

Massage is not a technique derived from one culture but from many. People the world over have used touch as a form of communication, comfort and defence throughout history. Animals also use touch in a similar way, for example grooming their young with their tongues or beaks, licking wounds after a fight and nuzzling or nudging each other to show affection. The following section provides a brief history of massage techniques and therapy.

THE ORIGINS AND HISTORY OF MASSAGE

What does 'massage' mean?

The word massage originates from many different languages. For example in Latin *massa* means 'that which forms a lump' and massage could be said to be a technique for removing the 'lumpiness' of the body, making it smooth. In Greek *massein* means 'to knead' and kneading is one of the fundamental movements used in this therapy. In French *masser* means 'to rub' and the basis of all massage is rubbing the skin and tissues. In Arabic *mass* means 'to touch or feel' which are both fundamental to massage.

The Ancients and massage

The use of massage has been recorded in China from 3000BC. The ancient Chinese called their technique 'amma', and used specific movements on particular points of the body. It was used for the promotion and restoration of health as well as for relaxation.

The Japanese also used the amma technique with similar pressure points but they called the points *tsubo*. Shiatsu — the application of pressure to certain points of the body in order to improve circulation, neural efficiency and general health — uses similar points and is a direct descendant of this ancient Japanese massage practice.

In India massage has always been used as part of traditional, Ayurvedic, medicine. The Ayurveda (from Sanskrit, *ayur* meaning life and *veda* knowledge) is an ancient medical text about the arts of healing and of prolonging life and it still forms the basis of much medical knowledge in India today.

All of these countries, both in the past and present, are renowned for their holistic, or whole body, mind and spirit approach to medicine. Massage is still used as a holistic treatment, considering the whole person not just the symptom or condition.

The Greeks

For the Ancient Greeks massage formed part of everyday exercise and fitness. Herodicus, fifth-century physician and teacher of Hippocrates, wrote about the benefits of massage and his student Hippocrates, known as the father of medicine, believed all doctors needed to know how to use massage for healing purposes.

The Romans

At the Roman baths, which were the site of everyday social and business life for all members of society, massage was central to the whole ritual. At Turkish baths, which are the closest modern-day equivalent to Roman baths, massage is still very important. In Roman times, massage was used for treating stiff and sore muscles and joints, curing disease, strengthening the constitution and improving circulation. Gladiators were given massage before and after their bouts of fighting. A physician named Galen, who was Greek but worked for the Roman Emperor, wrote many medical books stressing the use of massage for health purposes. And, of course, Julius Caesar, the renowned Roman emperor, had massage daily.

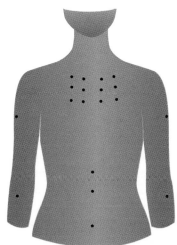

Shiatsu points on torso

THE HISTORY OF MASSAGE AND ITS USE

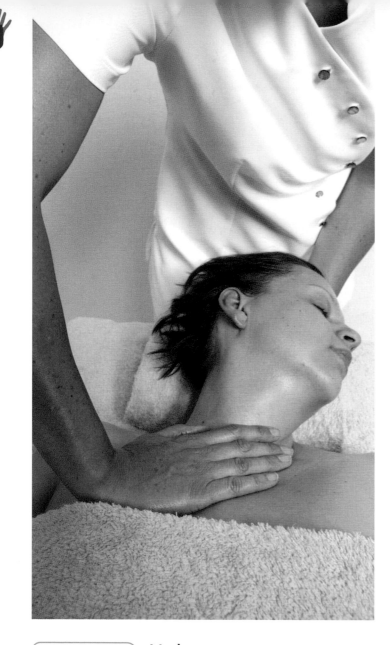

Facial massage

Modern massage

Modern massage is based on techniques developed by Per Henrik Ling (1776-1839), a physiologist and fencing master. He was from Sweden and massage is still referred to as Swedish massage because of his influence. In the eighteenth and nineteenth centuries, having studied in China, he developed a system of movements which he found helpful for improving his health and maintaining his physical condition. These movements are known as the Ling System and include techniques known as passive and active. His work was recognised first in his home country — in 1813 the Swedish government established the Royal Swedish Central Institute of Gymnastics of which Ling was named President — and subsequently around the world. In 1838 the Swedish Institute opened in London and there are now similar institutes in other countries.

Massage in the late nineteenth and early twentieth centuries

At the end of the nineteenth century massage was battling for respectability. The name was often used in relation to prostitution and therefore the therapy was not taken seriously. However, in order to combat this eight women founded The Society of Trained Masseuses in 1894. This later became the Chartered Society of Physiotherapy. Massage continued to be used extensively for medical purposes by doctors. In the two world wars massage was used to treat nerve injury and for rehabilitation. However, around this time mechanical methods of treatment began to replace manual methods. This led to a reduction in the use of therapeutic massage and a lack of awareness of its benefits.

Massage now

Massage has, in recent years, once again become a reputable and recognised therapy, thanks to an increased awareness of and interest in complementary therapies and alternative medicine. Many systems and methods exist but Swedish massage remains the basis for most practice. It can be used alone or in combination with other treatments and is a central part of therapies such as physiotherapy, stress-management and aromatherapy. Massage is beneficial to all body systems and is a natural and effective way to treat physical conditions.

You now know the origins of massage.

2 Anatomy for massage

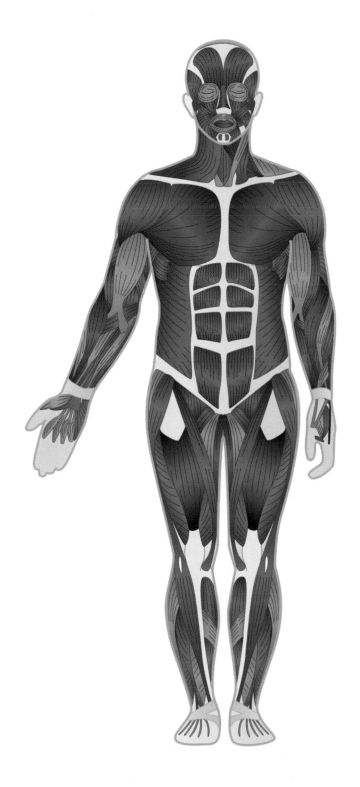

In Brief

Massage benefits the whole body, both physiologically and psychologically. However, some of the systems are more directly affected, particularly the skin, blood and lymph circulation, muscles and nerves. In order to understand how massage affects and benefits these systems it is useful to learn about their structure, their function and the diseases that affect them.

Learning objectives ●

The target knowledge of this chapter is:
● structure, function and diseases of the skin
● structure, function and diseases of the circulatory (vascular) system
● structure, function and diseases of the lymphatic system
● structure, function and diseases of the muscular system
● structure, function and diseases of the nervous system

THE SKIN

What is it?

The skin is the body's outer protective layer, also known as the integumentary system. It is the largest organ in the body, covering every part including the eyes, and varies in thickness. For example the skin on the soles of the feet is much thicker than the skin of the eyelids. There are two layers of skin, the epidermis and dermis or 'true skin', underneath which is the subcutaneous layer.

The epidermis is the skin that we see and is itself made up of layers of cells. The cells in the epidermis are constantly being desquamated (slowly rubbed off the body) and replaced. The dermis is the layer below the epidermis. This part of the skin contains blood, lymph and nerve vessels as well as sweat glands, sebaceous glands, hair follicles and living cells.

What does the skin do?

The skin has many functions:

- it secretes sebum, a natural moisturiser, from the sebaceous glands. Sebum lubricates the hair shafts, moisturises the skin and, combined with perspiration helps to form a barrier against bacteria called the acid mantle
- it helps regulate body temperature through vasodilation and vasoconstriction
- it waterproofs the body, although some substances can be absorbed, including certain drugs and essential oils
- it protects the body: its natural acid pH prevents bacterial invasion; melanin contained in the basal layer of the epidermis helps to protect the skin against damage from ultraviolet light

Cross-section of skin

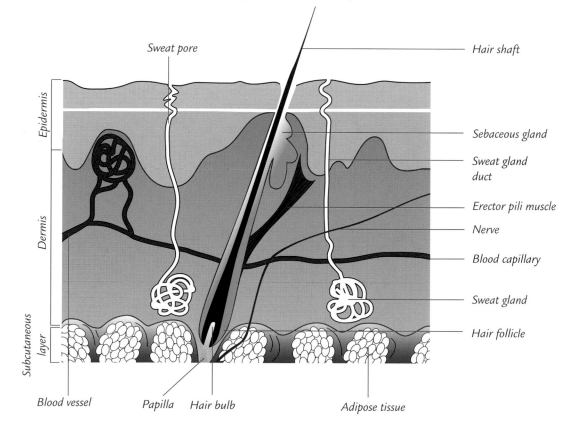

Sweat pore

Hair shaft

Epidermis

Dermis

Subcutaneous layer

Sebaceous gland

Sweat gland duct

Erector pili muscle

Nerve

Blood capillary

Sweat gland

Hair follicle

Blood vessel   Papilla   Hair bulb   Adipose tissue

- it eliminates waste through sweating
- it is the organ of touch, acting both as an information and warning system, telling the body about pain, pressure, heat and cold as well as the comfort and pleasure of contact
- it produces vitamin D, essential for the formation and maintenance of bone
- it produces melanin, the tanning pigment which darkens the skin in order to protect it from ultraviolet radiation.

Diseases of the skin

Massage therapists are in constant contact with the skin of their clients. It is therefore very important to be able to recognise skin conditions/diseases both for their own safety and that of the client.

Congenital conditions

These conditions may be inherited and often exist from birth.

- **Eczema**

The skin develops scaly, itchy, dry patches, sometimes with points of bleeding. It is found all over the body, but especially in the crook of the elbow, behind the knees, on the face, hands and scalp. It is not contagious. Not all forms of eczema are congenital. Atopic eczema occurs in people who may have an inherited tendency to allergy. Other forms of eczema (e.g. hand eczema) may be the result of irritation.

- **Psoriasis**

A chronic inflammation of the skin which causes red patches covered with silvery scales that are constantly shed. The size of the patches varies from minute points to whole limbs, with occasional bleeding. Psoriasis affects the whole body, particularly the knees, elbows, scalp, lower back and arms. It is not contagious.

- **Dermatitis**

Allergic reaction to substances that have either been taken in or come into contact with the skin. The skin is usually red and itchy and there may be tiny raised vesicles (blisters) which can burst, forming a dry crust which can crack and cause bleeding. This could cause a secondary infection.

Bacterial conditions

- **Acne rosacea**

This is an eruption which affects the face, nose and cheeks. It has a red, flushed appearance and may be lumpy and thick with possible pustules. It can be associated with the menopause or other hormonal changes, therefore it is more common in women than men. It is aggravated by hot, spicy foods, caffeine, alcohol and changes in temperature. Not contagious.

- **Acne vulgaris**

The skin develops papules, pustules and comedones and has a shiny, sallow appearance. Acne vulgaris may be caused by hormonal imbalances, particularly in puberty, resulting in over-active sebaceous glands. The excess of sebum blocks the pores and causes infection. It mainly affects the face, back, chest and shoulders. Although not contagious, acne vulgaris is contraindicated because touching the affected area can spread the condition or burst pustules.

- **Boils**

An infection which causes inflammation around a hair follicle. Avoid touching the area during massage.

- **Folliculitis**

An infection of the sebaceous gland and hair follicle which causes inflammation and often occurs in conjunction with acne vulgaris. Avoid touching during massage. Common on buttocks, thigh, neck and armpits.

- **Impetigo**
A highly contagious infection which causes blisters which weep and develop a thick, yellow crust. Common around the nose and mouth. Contraindicated.

Viral conditions

Massage is contraindicated for these viral conditions because they are highly contagious.

- **Herpes simplex**
Herpes simplex is commonly known as a cold sore. It causes small blisters which usually occur on the mouth but can spread to other parts of the body. The blisters eventually dry up forming a crust which falls off. Contagious.

- **Herpes zoster**
This viral infection is commonly known as shingles and is the adult form of chicken pox. It is a nervous system disorder, usually affecting the spinal nerves and one side of the thorax and causes a rash of blisters with very severe itching. Highly contagious.

- **Warts**
Growths on the skin, of which there are many types. Avoid the area.

- **Verrucas**
Warts found on the feet. Avoid the area.

Fungal conditions

Fungal conditions are infections which attach themselves mainly to keratinised structures such as the skin. Massage is contraindicated for fungal conditions which are highly infectious.

- **Tinea corporis**
This is also known as ringworm and is found all over the body.

- **Tinea pedis**
This is commonly known as athlete's foot and is found on the feet.

Other

- **Allergic reactions including urticaria**
When the skin is irritated it produces histamine as a defence. This can cause watery, stinging eyes, itching, swellings, red blotchy patches and a runny nose. Urticaria (also known as nettle rash or hives) is a severe allergic reaction characterised by pinkish weals. Therapists should ensure at consultation stage that the client has no allergies that may be provoked by massage or the medium used.

- **Skin cancer**
Skin cancer is caused by excessive exposure to sunlight and contraindicated for massage because of the risk of spreading it.

- **Basal cell carcinoma**
The skin develops nodules or shallow ulcers with raised edges. It occurs on exposed parts of the skin, especially face, nose, eyelid, cheek and is the least malignant skin cancer.

- **Squamous cell carcinoma**
Squamous cells are the type of cell found on the top layer of the skin. This cancer consists of a swelling, that may resemble a wart or ulcer, that grows rapidly.

- **Malignant melanoma**
A malignant tumour of melanocytes (the cells that produce melanin). It usually develops in a previously benign mole. The mole may become larger and darker, and may itch or bleed. The tumour eventually spreads. This is the most malignant skin cancer.

You now know what the skin is, what it does and the types of diseases that affect it.

THE CIRCULATORY (VASCULAR) SYSTEM

What is it?

The circulatory system is the body's transport system, composed of the heart, blood and blood vessels. Blood carries the body's fuel and the heart is the body's engine. The heart pumps blood around the body in a system of vessels known as arteries, veins and capillaries.

Arteries carry oxygenated (arterial) blood from the heart and veins carry deoxygenated (venous) blood back to the heart. Capillaries are tiny porous vessels at the end of the arteries which distribute oxygen, nutrients and fluid and collect carbon dioxide, waste and fluid.

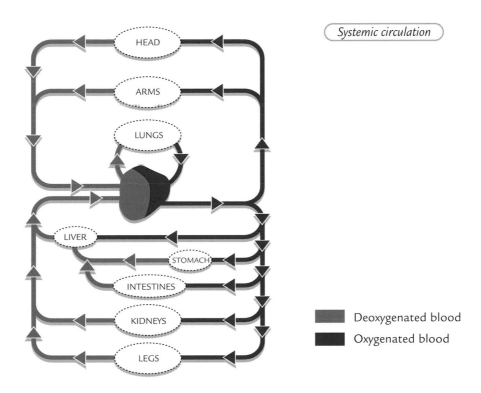

Systemic circulation

HEAD

ARMS

LUNGS

LIVER

STOMACH

INTESTINES

KIDNEYS

LEGS

■ Deoxygenated blood
■ Oxygenated blood

What does it do?

It pumps and transports blood, a fluid connective tissue consisting of different types of cells which is used to distribute nutrients and oxygen to the tissues, and waste and carbon dioxide from the tissues. Blood also carries hormones and contains cells that help fight infection (leucocytes). It also transports heat and therefore helps with heat regulation.

Diseases of the circulatory system

Massage stimulates the circulation so any circulatory disorders may be aggravated by it. The therapist should ensure that the client has no contra-indicated circulatory diseases at the consultation stage and contact the client's GP if in any doubt about the suitability of treatment.

Anaemia

Anaemia is a reduction in the blood's ability to carry oxygen, caused either by a decrease in red blood cells, or the haemoglobin they carry, or both. It may be caused by extensive loss of blood, lack of iron in the diet, the failure of bone marrow to produce the normal level of cells or it may be inherited.

Arteriosclerosis

A degenerative disease of the arteries, in which the walls of the vessels harden and lose elasticity. The loss of elasticity causes an increase in blood pressure. This condition mainly affects the elderly.

Atherosclerosis

A build-up of fats, including cholesterol, inside the arteries which causes a narrowing of the artery passage, hardening of the vessel walls and a loss of elasticity.

Haemophilia

The blood's inability to clot. This is an inherited disease which affects mainly men but which can be carried by women.

Haemorrhoids

Also known as piles, these are enlarged veins in the rectum or anus which may collapse or contain blood clots.

Heart conditions

Any client with a history of heart disease, angina or heart attacks should have treatment approved by a GP.

Hepatitis A B C

Inflammations of the liver, caused by viruses, toxic substances or immunological abnormalities. Type A is spread by fecally contaminated food. Types B and C are transmitted by infected body fluids including blood. Contagious.

High blood pressure

High blood pressure (hypertension) is blood pressure that consistently remains above the normal level. It is caused by many different factors including stress, poor diet, smoking and obesity. Stimulating massage may aggravate this condition because it invigorates the circulation. If the client suffers from hypertension, the therapist will need to check with the GP that massage is safe as the client may be taking medication for their condition that might result in fluctuations in blood pressure.

High cholesterol

High cholesterol is an excessive build-up of a fatty substance called cholesterol, which can cause a reduction in arterial capacity (atherosclerosis – see previous page) and thus high blood pressure.

Leukaemia

Leukaemia is a cancer of the blood, caused by over-production of white blood cells.

Low blood pressure

Low blood pressure (hypotension) is blood pressure that consistently remains below the normal level. It is not usually contraindicated for massage unless severe, in which case the GP should be consulted and then, if safe, the therapist should carry out a gentle massage as even with gentle massage blood pressure will drop once the parasympathetic nervous system is stimulated.

Phlebitis

Inflammation of a vein. Thrombo-phlebitis is the inflammation of a vein where a blood clot has formed.

Stress

Stress can be defined as any factor which affects mental or physical health. When a person is stressed, the heart beats faster, thus pumping blood more quickly. Excessive and unresolved stress can lead to high blood pressure, coronary thrombosis and heart attacks.

Thrombosis

A blood clot in a blood vessel. Always contraindicated because massage may move it and cause further complications.

Varicose veins

Varicose veins are caused by the collapse of valves in veins and are commonly found in the lower legs. Venous blood has to travel uphill in order to return to the heart and valves in the veins help prevent backward flow. Sometimes these valves no longer work effectively and the venous blood collects, dilating and distending the veins, creating bluish knobbly veins. Massage should only be used above and not directly on varicose veins as this may weaken them further and can be very painful for the client.

You now know what the circulatory system is, what it does and the types of diseases that affect it.

THE LYMPHATIC SYSTEM

What is it?

The lymphatic system is a secondary circulation which is intertwined with and supports the blood. It consists of lymphatic vessels, lymph nodes, lymphatic ducts and lymph.

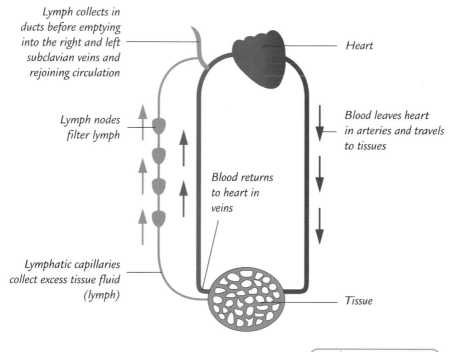

Lymph collects in ducts before emptying into the right and left subclavian veins and rejoining circulation

Heart

Lymph nodes filter lymph

Blood leaves heart in arteries and travels to tissues

Blood returns to heart in veins

Lymphatic capillaries collect excess tissue fluid (lymph)

Tissue

Lymph circuit (simplified)

What does it do?

The lymphatic system drains excess tissue fluid from the spaces around tissues, rather than from the tissues themselves. Excess fluid and large particles in the tissue spaces that cannot pass back through the small pores of the capillaries are collected by lymphatic capillaries. They transport this fluid, known as lymph, to lymph vessels and then to lymph nodes which filter it to remove any waste, toxins or bacteria. The lymphatic system also protects against infection and disease by producing antibodies and white blood cells, known as lymphocytes, in lymph nodes. These protective cells are added to the lymph before it is returned to the circulation.

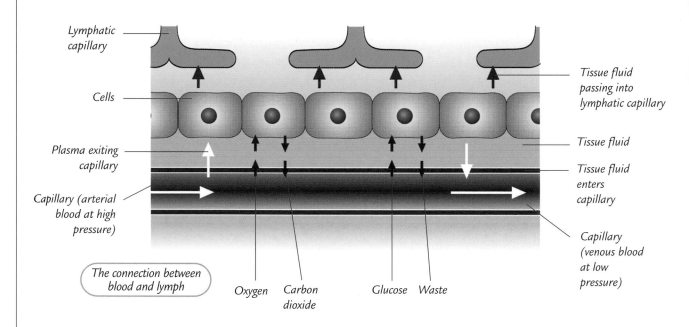

Lymphatic capillary

Cells

Plasma exiting capillary

Capillary (arterial blood at high pressure)

The connection between blood and lymph

Oxygen   Carbon dioxide   Glucose   Waste

Tissue fluid passing into lymphatic capillary

Tissue fluid

Tissue fluid enters capillary

Capillary (venous blood at low pressure)

Diseases and disorders of the lymphatic system

Massage improves lymphatic circulation. Any fever or infection is contraindicated not only because it is unsafe for the therapist but also because it may be spread by the treatment.

Lymphoedema

Lymphoedema is a form of swelling caused by a malfunction of the lymphatic system. It is caused by poor drainage either because the lymph vessels have been damaged or the lymph has become trapped. As with varicose veins poor lymph drainage can start a cycle: once lymph gets trapped and collects it then sits in the vessel stretching and distending it which causes poor drainage. Lymphoedema usually affects the arms or legs. Massage, particularly lymphatic drainage massage, can be very beneficial. See Chapter 7 for more details.

Hodgkin's Lymphoma

Cancer of the lymphoid tissue. The lymphatic nodes swell painlessly, either in one area or several. Other symptoms include weight loss, weakness, itchiness, fever, anaemia and lowered immunity. Contraindicated.

You now know what the lymphatic system is, what it does and the types of diseases that affect it.

THE MUSCULAR SYSTEM

What is the muscular system?

The muscular system consists of muscles and their attachments, known as tendons and fascia, which connect the muscles to bones and joints. There are three types of muscle, cardiac, involuntary and voluntary. Cardiac muscle is only found in the heart and works to pump blood around the body. Involuntary (smooth) muscles are the muscles that we do not consciously control, such as those in the walls of blood vessels. Voluntary (skeletal) muscles are the muscles that we consciously control, such as those in our arms and legs.

What does the muscular system do?

The muscular system enables movement. Muscles consist of muscle fibres and when these fibres contract the muscle changes shape and moves the part of the body to which it is attached. Muscles also stabilise the joints, help control body temperature through shivering and dilation of the capillaries and maintain postural tone. At any one time, however relaxed we might think we are, there are muscles contracting in order for us to sit, stand or lie down.

Why is it important to know about muscles for massage?

Throughout a massage, the therapist's movements are working over muscles and it is very important to know which voluntary muscles are being treated at any time, what they do (their action) and how the massage may affect them. Voluntary or skeletal muscles usually have two ends, known as the origin (part closest to the midline/body and the part which is the fixed end of the muscle and therefore hardly moves) and the insertion (part furthest away from midline and the moving end of the muscle). Muscles always work from their insertion to their origin and when massaging, movements are usually carried out in the direction of the heart, therefore from the insertion towards the origin. It is important to understand the position of the muscles as shown in the diagrams on the preceding pages and their action. The following table (page 22) details the origin, insertion and action of the major muscles of the body.

Diseases of the muscular system

Massage movements directly affect the muscles and are generally beneficial for most conditions affecting them.

Atony

Lack of normal tone or tension in a muscle.

Atrophy

Caused by ndernourishmentor lack of use. The effects are wasting away, or failure to reach normal size, of bulk of muscle.

Cramp

Cramp is a sustained involuntary contraction of a muscle, perhaps caused by salt deficiency. Massage is one of the most effective ways of relieving cramp.

Fibrositis

Build-up of lactic acid inside the muscles causing inflammation of tissues, stiffness and pain. Lumbago is a form of fibrositis of the muscles in the lumbar area of the back. Torticollis, or 'wry neck' is a form of fibrositis of the sternocleidomastoid muscle in the neck which causes the head to lean to one side.

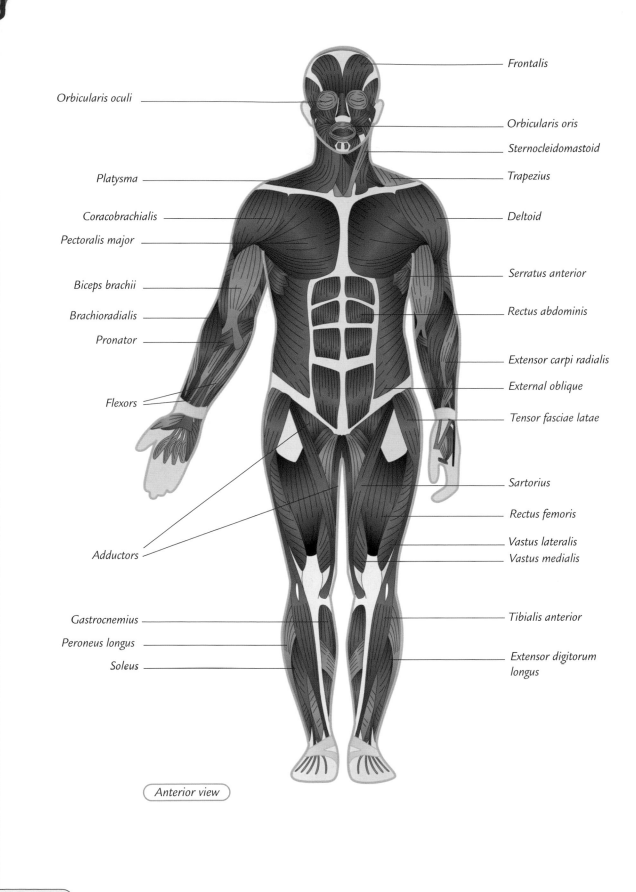

Frontalis

Orbicularis oculi

Orbicularis oris

Sternocleidomastoid

Trapezius

Platysma

Coracobrachialis

Deltoid

Pectoralis major

Serratus anterior

Biceps brachii

Rectus abdominis

Brachioradialis

Pronator

Extensor carpi radialis

External oblique

Tensor fasciae latae

Flexors

Sartorius

Rectus femoris

Vastus lateralis

Vastus medialis

Adductors

Gastrocnemius

Tibialis anterior

Peroneus longus

Soleus

Extensor digitorum longus

Anterior view

MASSAGE

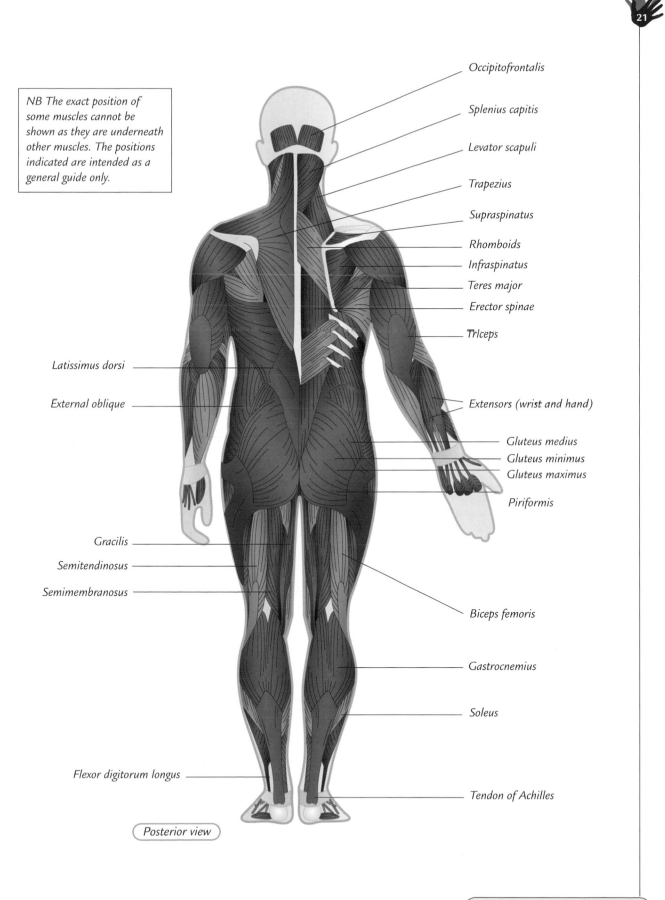

NB The exact position of some muscles cannot be shown as they are underneath other muscles. The positions indicated are intended as a general guide only.

Occipitofrontalis

Splenius capitis

Levator scapuli

Trapezius

Supraspinatus

Rhomboids

Infraspinatus

Teres major

Erector spinae

Trlceps

Latissimus dorsi

External oblique

Extensors (wrist and hand)

Gluteus medius

Gluteus minimus

Gluteus maximus

Piriformis

Gracilis

Semitendinosus

Semimembranosus

Biceps femoris

Gastrocnemius

Soleus

Flexor digitorum longus

Tendon of Achilles

Posterior view

Muscles of the torso	Origin	Insertion	Main actions
Sternocleidomastoid	Sternum & clavicle	Mastoid process	One side only – flexes neck laterally and rotates it Both – side flexion
Scalenes	Transverse processes of 2nd to 6th cervical	Upper surfaces of ribs 1 and 2	Raises first two ribs, flexes and rotates the neck
Splenius capitis	First six thoracic vertebrae	Mastoid process and occipital bone	Extends the neck Slight rotation
Levator scapulae	Upper four cervical vertebrae	Superior medial border of scapula	Elevates shoulder, rotates scapula
Supraspinatus	Supraspinous fossa of scapula	Greater tuberosity of humerus	Abducts arm
Infraspinatus	Inferior spinous fossa of scapula	Greater tuberosity of humerus	Rotates arm outwards (laterally)
Subscapularis	Subscapular fossa of scapula	Lesser tuberosity of humerus	Rotates arm inwards
Teres minor	Axillary border of scapula	Greater tuberosity of humerus	Rotates arm outwards (laterally)
Teres major	Inferior angle of scapula	Medial lip of bicipital groove of humerus	Draws arm backwards, adducts and medially rotates it
Rhomboid major & minor	7th cervical and 1st to 5th thoracic vertebrae	Medial border of scapula	Adducts (draws towards spine) and rotates scapula downwards
Trapezius	Occipital bone, cervical and thoracic vertebrae	Clavicle and spine of scapula Acromion process	Elevates and braces shoulder, rotates scapula
Latissimus dorsi	Lower six thoracic and lumbar vertebrae Sacrum and illiac crest	Bicipital groove of humerus	Draws arm backwards, adducts and rotates it inwards
Erector spinae	Sacrum and iliac crest, ribs and lower vertebrae	Ribs, vertebrae and mastoid process,	One side only – flexes trunk laterally Both – extends trunk
Quadratus lumborum	Iliac crest	12th rib and transverse processes of upper four lumbar vertebrae	One side only – flexes trunk laterally and rotates it Both – extends trunk
Pectoralis major	Clavicle, sternum, upper six costal cartilages	Lateral lip of bicipital groove of humerus	Draws arm forwards (flexes) and adducts and rotates it inwards (medial rotation)
Pectoralis minor	3rd to 5th ribs	Coracoid process of scapula	Draws shoulder forwards and downwards
Serratus anterior	Upper nine ribs	Anterior surface of vertebral border of scapula	Draws shoulder forwards and rotates scapula
Rectus abdominus	Pubis	Ribs and sternum	Flexes the trunk
Abdominus tranversalis	Inguinal ligament, iliac crest, lumbar fascia, cartilages of lower six ribs	Conjoint tendon and linea alba through abdominal aponeurosis, pubis	Supports the viscera, compresses abdomen

Muscles of the torso (cont)	Origin	Insertion	Main actions
Internal obliques	Inguinal ligament, iliac crest and lumbar fascia	Costal cartilages of ribs 9–12 and linea alba	Lumbar flexion, side flexion and rotation
External obliques	Lower eight ribs	Iliac crest and linea alba through abdominal aponeurosis	Lumbar flexion, side flexion and rotation
Muscles of the arm			
Deltoid	Clavicle, acromion process and spine of scapula	Deltoid tuberosity of humerus	Front draws arm forwards Middle abducts the arm Back draws arm backwards
Coracobrachialis	Coracoid process of scapula	Shaft of humerus	Adducts and flexes the arm, horizontally adducts the shoulder
Biceps brachii	Long head – supra glenoid tubercle of scapula Short head – coracoid process of scapula	Tuberosity of radius	Flexes elbow, supinates forearm
Brachialis	Shaft of humerus	Coronoid process of ulna	Flexes elbow
Brachioradialis	Lateral condyloid ridge of humerus	Distal part of radius	Flexes elbow
Triceps brachii	Long head – scapula Medial head – humerus Lateral head – humerus	Olecranon process of ulna	Extends elbow
Anconeus	Lateral epicondyle of humerus	Olecranon process of ulna	Extends elbow
Pronator teres	Above medial epicondyle of humerus and coronoid process of ulna	Middle of shaft of radius	Pronates forearm and hand
Supinator	Lateral epicondyle of humerus	Lateral surface of radius	Supinates forearm and hand
Extensor digitorum	Lateral epicondyle of humerus	Metacarpals and phalanges	Extends wrist and fingers
Extensor carpi radialis brevis & longus	Lateral epicondyle of humerus	2nd and 3rd metacarpals	Extends and abducts wrist
Extensor carpi ulnaris	Lateral epicondyle of humerus	5th metacarpal	Extends wrist
Flexor carpi radialis	Medial epicondyle of humerus	2nd and 3rd metacarpals	Flexes wrist
Flexor carpi ulnaris	Medial epicondyle of humerus and ulna	5th metatcarpal, pisiform and hamate	Flexes wrist
Muscles of the leg			
Iliopsoas Psoas Iliacus	12th thoracic and all lumbar vertebrae, iliac fossa and front of sacrum	Lesser trochanter of femur	Flexes the thigh and laterally rotates femur
Gluteus maximus	Posterior crest of ilium, posterior surface of sacrum and coccyx	Gluteal tuberosity of femur	Tenses fascia lata and extends hip, raises trunk after stooping

Muscles of the leg (cont)	Origin	Insertion	Main actions
Gluteus medius	Posterior surface of ilium	Greater trochanter of femur	Abducts and medially rotates femur
Gluteus minimus	Lateral surface of ilium	Greater trochanter of femur	Abducts and medially rotates femur
Piriformis	Front of sacrum	Greater trochanter of femur	Laterally rotates femur
Tensor fascia lata	Anterior iliac crest	Fascia lata	Abducts and rotates the femur
Biceps femoris	Long head – ischium Short head – linea aspera	Head of fibula and lateral condyle of tibia	Extends hip, flexes knee
Semimembranosus	Ischial tuberosity	Medial condyle of tibia	Extends hip, flexes knee
Semitendinosus	Ischial tuberosity	Below medial condyle of tibia	Extends hip, flexes knee
Rectus femoris	Above acetabulum	Through patella and patellar tendon on to tibial tuberosity	Extends knee, flexes hip
Vastus lateralis	Greater trochanter and linea aspera	Through patella and patellar tendon on to tibial tuberosity	Extends knee
Vastus intermedius	Shaft of femur	Through patella and patellar tendon on to tibial tuberosity	Extends knee
Vastus medialis	Whole length of linea aspera	Through patella and patellar tendon on to tibial tuberosity	Extends knee
Sartorius	Anterior superior iliac spine	Below medial condyle of tibia	Flexes, abducts and rotates femur laterally, flexes knee
Gracilis	Pubis and ischium	Below medial condyle of tibia	Adducts and medially rotates femur, flexes knee
Adductors – longus, brevis & magnus	Pubis and ischium	Linea aspera and supra-condylar line	Adducts femur
Pectineus	Pubis	Close to lesser trochanter of femur	Adducts femur, flexes hip
Popliteus	Lateral condyle of femur	Tibia	Internally rotates and flexes the knee
Gastrocnemius	Medial and lateral condyles of femur	Through Achilles tendon to calcaneum	Plantarflexes the foot, flexes the knee
Soleus	Fibula and tibia	Calcaneum	Plantarflexes the foot
Peroneus longus	Fibula	Medial cuneiform and 1st metatarsal	Everts foot and plantarflexes ankle
Peroneus brevis	Fibula	5th metatarsal	Plantarflexes the ankle
Tibialis anterior	Shaft of tibia	Medial cuneiform and 1st metatarsal	Dorsiflexes and inverts the foot
Tibialis posterior	Tibia and fibula	Navicular and 2nd to 4th metatarsals	Inverts and plantarflexes the foot
Extensor digitorum longus	Tibia and fibula	Distal phalanges of toes	Extends toes, dorsiflexes the ankle and everts foot
Flexor digitorum longus	Posterior of tibia	Distal phalanges of toes	Flexes toes, plantarflexes the ankle and inverts foot

Myositis
Inflammation of a muscle.

Rupture
Burst or tear in the fascia or sheath surrounding muscles.

Spasm
A more than usual number of muscle fibres in sustained contraction, usually in response to pain. Fibres contract for much longer than is usually necessary.

Spasticity
This is caused when inhibitory nerves have been cut. Its effects are that spinal reflexes cause sustained contraction.

Sprain
A sudden twist or wrench of the joint's ligaments.

Strain
An over-stretching of a muscle, causing soreness and localised pain. May sometimes indicate a rupture (tear) in muscle fibres, tendon or fascia.

Stress
Stress is any factor which affects physical or mental well-being. Its effects are excessive muscle tension and subsequent muscle pain, especially in the back and neck.

You now know what the muscular system is, what it does and the types of diseases that affect it.

THE NERVOUS SYSTEM

What is it?

The nervous system is a communication and instruction network. It consists of two parts: the central nervous system (brain and spinal cord) and the peripheral nervous system (cranial nerves, spinal nerves, autonomic system including the parasympathetic and sympathetic nervous systems). The central nervous system controls the functions of the mind and behaviour as well as interpreting and reacting to the peripheral nervous system's messages; the peripheral nervous system controls our motor and sensory functions plus the action of the internal organs and sends information relating to them back to the brain.

What does it do?

The nervous system is one of the body's communication and instruction networks. The brain is the centre and it is connected to the rest of the body by nerve cells which carry information and instructions to and from it. When the brain is informed of danger, sensation or pain it can protect the body by sending out a warning. Thus, when a finger is placed in very hot water, the nerves send a message to the brain telling it that the water is too hot and may burn the skin and the brain sends a message telling the finger to move. We do not perceive this process because nerve impulses are involuntary and extremely fast.

Diseases of the nervous system

The nervous system can be stimulated by massage. Sufferers of severe nervous pain may find massage too painful and counterproductive over the affected areas but massage of related areas may be appropriate. Clients suffering from stress or mild nervous conditions may find it extremely helpful.

Bell's palsy

Facial paralysis, caused by injury to or infection of the facial nerve which subsequently becomes inflamed.

Motor neurone disease

A rare progressive disorder, in which the motor neurones in the body gradually deteriorate structurally and functionally.

Parkinson's disease

Progressive disease caused by damage to basal ganglia of the brain and resulting in loss of dopamine (neuro-transmitter). Causes tremor and rigidity in muscles, as well as difficulty and slowness with voluntary movement.

Stress

Such factors can be imagined, (e.g. worry about the future) or real, (e.g. financial problems). It is not the factor itself that is damaging but the response to it. Stress puts all the systems of the body on red alert, particularly the nervous system which tries to locate the danger, whether real or not, in order to tell the brain. This heightened activity causes symptoms such as churning stomach or 'butterflies', racing heart or palpitations, diarrhoea, loss of appetite, trembling, insomnia and sweating. Massage is extremely effective for treating stress because it stimulates the parasympathetic nervous system which slows down the action of some internal organs, particularly the heart.

Sciatica

Sciatica is often caused by the degeneration of an intervertebral disc which then causes pain in the lower back and the outside of the leg and foot. Massage is contraindicated over the affected area but soothing massage of the upper body may help relaxation and provide some pain relief.

Neuralgia
Stabbing pain along one or more nerves. Massage may be too painful over the affected area. Massage may also trigger neuralgia, which can be affected by light touch.

Neuritis
Inflammation of a nerve causing severe pain along it. Massage would be too painful over the affected area.

Myalgic encephalomyelitis (ME)
ME is also known as post-viral fatigue. Symptoms and suspected causes vary. It is characterised by extreme exhaustion which cannot be relieved by sleep or rest, general aches and pains, headaches and sometimes sore throat, fever, depression and swollen lymph nodes. Massage can sometimes provide a much needed dose of deep relaxation as well as an increased sense of well-being. It can also exhaust sufferers.

Multiple sclerosis
A disease which causes loss of the protective myelin sheath from nerve fibres in the central nervous system. Sufferers lose muscular coordination, sensation and have problems with speech and vision. Massage can help prevent spasm and stiffness in the muscles but the client should be referred before treatment.

You now know the basic structure and function of the skin, blood and lymph circulation, muscles and nerves and some of the diseases which affect them.

SUMMARY
- *Massage is used over the whole surface of the body but is particularly beneficial for the circulation, skin, muscles and joints.*

50% OFF
FULL ACCESS

DON'T FORGET NOW YOU CAN USE A RANGE OF ONLINE LEARNING RESOURCES FOR JUST £10 (NORMAL RRP £20)

The Massage e-Learning Resource has been designed to enhance your learning experience

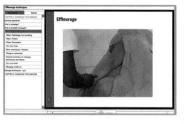

☐ Bring knowledge to life with videos of each technique as well as a full massage routine

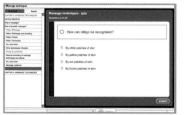

☐ Manage your learning with step-by-step modules and integrated 'classroom' sessions

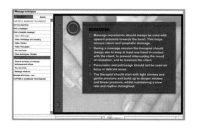

☐ Absorb information on key topics with interactive exercises and learning activities

To login to use these **e-learning resources**, visit **www.emspublishing.co.uk/massage** and follow the onscreen instructions

AN INTRODUCTORY GUIDE TO

Massage

3 Massage techniques

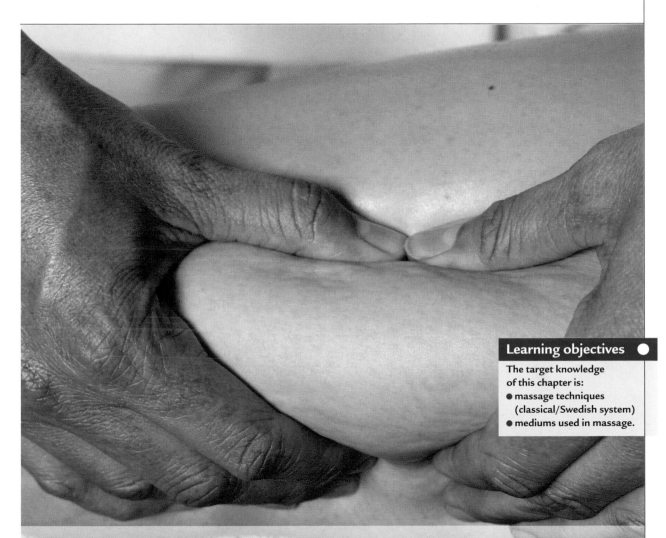

Learning objectives

The target knowledge
of this chapter is:
- massage techniques
  (classical/Swedish system)
- mediums used in massage.

In Brief

Massage is the manipulation of the soft tissues of the body, leading to benefits for all the body systems. The techniques in this book, which are based on the Swedish system, use the application of pressure to either soothe or stimulate.

MASSAGE TECHNIQUES

What is massage?
Massage is a combination of various movements used to manipulate tissues for both local and overall effects and benefits. The movements range from gentle stroking to invigorating friction, depending on the desired effect. Massage is generally based on the Swedish system and several types of massage have developed which incorporate these techniques for different therapeutic effects.

What is Swedish massage?
The Swedish system of massage is named after the man who developed it, Per Henrik Ling. He was a physiologist and fencing master and developed a system of movements which he found helpful for improving his health and maintaining his physical condition. Classical massage is still based on the techniques he used, i.e. effleurage, petrissage and percussion. This chapter will look at these fundamental movements as well as variations of them.

EFFLEURAGE

What is effleurage?
The name effleurage derives from *effleurer*, a French word meaning 'to touch lightly'. It is generally a gentle, sweeping, relaxing stroke, with varying levels of pressure, used at the beginning and end of a massage. It can also be used with firm pressure over large areas once the muscles are relaxed. Unlike petrissage and percussion, effleurage does not aim to move or manipulate tissues or muscles, only to soothe and relax them and improve circulation.

Effleurage

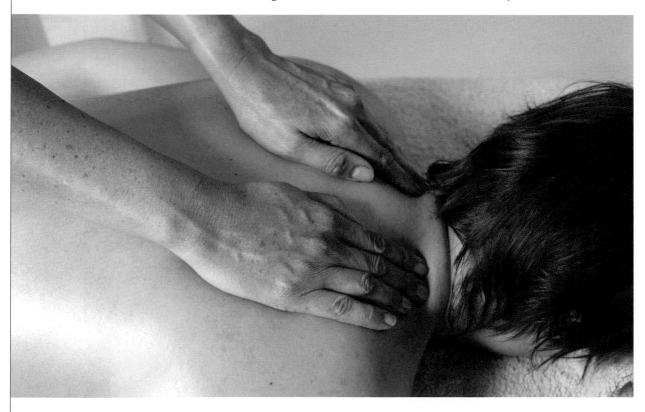

How to do it

With fingers and thumbs together, keep the hands relaxed and stroke the skin slowly and rhythmically with a confident pressure. When massaging the limbs, the emphasis of the pressure is towards the heart. The hands may be used one after the other or at the same time. The whole palm of the hand and the fingers should be used to prevent tickling the client. Hands must mould to the contours of the area being treated. Once a gentle rhythm has been established the therapist can increase the pressure gradually to prepare the body for the deeper work that follows.

If you remember only one thing...

Effleurage is a relaxing stroke that is used to prepare the body for deeper techniques.

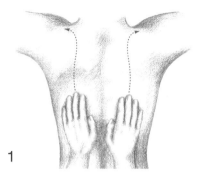

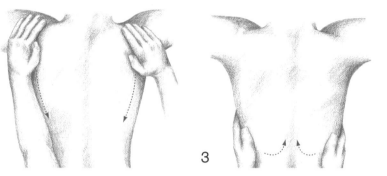

1   2   3

When to use it

Effleurage is used at the start and finish of a massage session and at the start and finish of each body part, e.g. at the beginning and end of work on the back or legs. It is also used as a connection stroke between different parts of the massage. When carrying out a massage the therapist must not break contact with the client because when the hands are removed the client's body senses this, believes the massage is over and begins to rouse itself from its relaxed state.

return of blood to the heart and aids lymph drainage. Deep effleurage also pushes blood into superficial capillaries.

The three stages of effleurage (on the back)

What does it do?

As the first contact between therapist and client, effleurage helps to prepare the body for massage, introducing the client to the therapist's touch, spreading the massage medium such as oil or cream (if used), warming the skin and relaxing the client. It is also used after more invigorating strokes to help the elimination of toxins from the areas that have been worked. It can also help desquamation, especially when used deeply, and thus help the skin to regenerate. Effleurage on the limbs with the pressure working towards the heart assists the

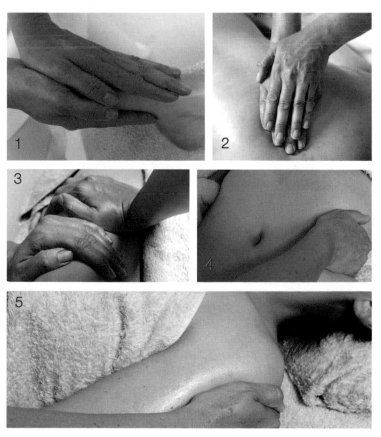

MASSAGE TECHNIQUES

PETRISSAGE

What is petrissage?

Petrissage, like effleurage, is a name derived from French. *Pétrir* means to knead or rub with force and this stroke uses both kneading and rubbing movements to manipulate tissues and muscles. It uses the pressure of the hands or fingers to break down tension. There are various methods: in some cases only the fingers and/or thumbs are used to knead the tissues, in others the whole hand is used.

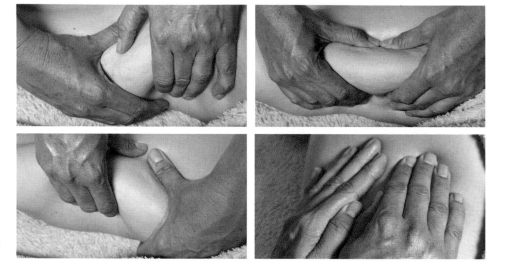

Kneading is a petrissage stroke

KNEADING

Carefully and slowly grasp the flesh of the part of the body being worked with both hands or fingers then use one hand to lift it, as if pulling it away from the bone. Keep the tissues firmly compressed whilst lifting, then release and repeat with the other hand. Continue to lift, compress and release with alternate hands, as if kneading dough and build up into a rhythm. For particularly stiff/tight areas, build a twist into the movement so that the flesh is being 'wrung' like a damp cloth. The pressure should be smooth and not jerky and care should be taken to avoid pinching the skin. Begin gently and build up to firmer pressure, always using the same rate and rhythm and getting feedback from the client. It is important to use body weight and movement to assist in making the technique effective and less tiring for the therapist. Lean into the muscle as you grasp it and lean back as you lift.

When to use it

Petrissage usually follows effleurage at the start of a massage. It should be used to break down tightness and tension in large muscles. It should not be used on bony or delicate areas.

What does it do?

Kneading stretches the muscles, and compresses tissue against tissue improving suppleness and elasticity, and helps break down tension and stiffness in tissues and large muscles. Such stiffness is often caused by the build-up of toxins such as lactic acid. Kneading helps to release and break down these toxins, enabling the muscles to work more efficiently.

If you remember only one thing...

Petrissage (or kneading) is a firm application of pressure which compresses tissue against tissue, thus releasing muscle tightness and breaking down toxins and tension.

MASSAGE

FRICTION

It also stimulates the circulation. Despite the firmness of the stroke it is more relaxing than invigorating because it releases any tight muscles and the toxins within. The name friction, like many others used in massage, comes from a Latin word, *fricare*, which means to rub or rub down. Friction techniques are all variations of rubbing and they work by compressing tissue against bone. It is often used for close work on a small area or on specific areas of tightness.

How to do it

Place thumbs or fingers, particularly the balls/pads of the thumb, on the section of the body to be worked. Apply firm pressure from your body and circle the tissue immediately below the thumbs slowly and deeply. Try to imagine the tissues below the surface of the skin and how the rubbing movement pushes them against other muscles and against the bones creating friction. The thumbs can be rubbed up and down or held in a static position. Fingertips can also be used if the therapist finds them more effective. Once the small area has been thoroughly worked move to another section. The therapist should not be moving rapidly across an expanse of flesh but deliberately and slowly focusing on a small section at a time, moving along the length of a muscle. Depending on the type of skin/ individual's requirements the therapist will need to adjust the length of time spent on each small area in order to prevent rubbing for too long and causing soreness. The effect should be one of heat and tension.

Cross-fibre friction is a variation of this technique in which the therapist works across the muscle at right angles to the fibres instead of along the length of the muscle. This helps to stretch the muscle fibres and release tension. It is used extensively by physiotherapists and sports massage therapists in the treatment of injuries.

When to use it

Friction is a method used for focusing on a particular problem area. It is especially useful for releasing tension in muscles and for loosening tightness around joints. It is not recommended for use all over the body because it is time-consuming and tiring for the therapist. It is also used on small muscles where petrissage is not appropriate. On tight muscles friction can be very painful, so caution is vital in the care of the client.

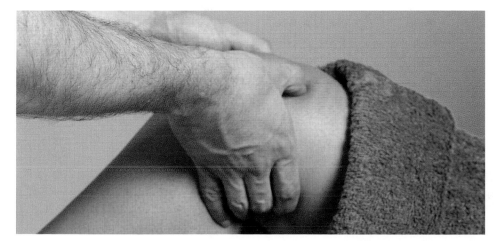

FRICTION

Frictions are firm rubbing and heat-producing techniques which compress tissue against bone. They are used for close work on areas of tension or by physiotherapists or sports massage therapists in treating injury.

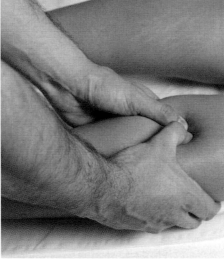

What does it do?

Friction movements heat up the local area, improve circulation, promote lymph drainage, stimulate the nerves and loosen tightness in the muscles. Working very closely with the muscles helps to break down any local 'knottiness' or lumpiness. Cross-fibre friction helps stretch the muscle fibres and release any tension held in the muscle; it also allows the therapist, particularly in sports massage, to work close to a damaged or inflamed area without touching it, because working on one section of muscle helps stretch the rest of the muscle.

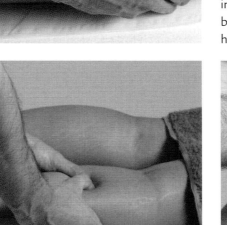

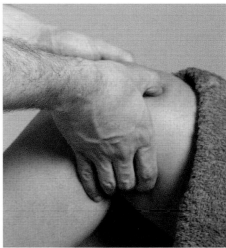

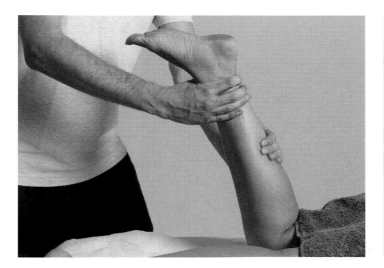

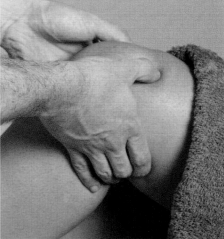

PERCUSSION

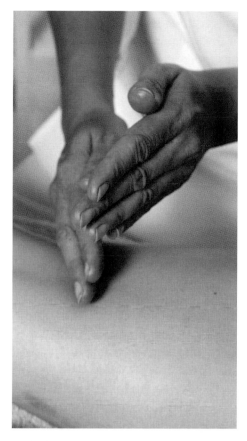

What is percussion?

Percussion derives from the Latin word *percutere* meaning to hit. Percussion techniques are brisk, invigorating and stimulating strokes, which use the hands to strike the body rapidly and suddenly. The classic 'chopping' motion associated with Swedish massage is a percussion technique called hacking. The others are pounding, beating, cupping and tapotement.

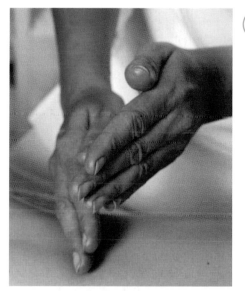

A classic massage technique called hacking

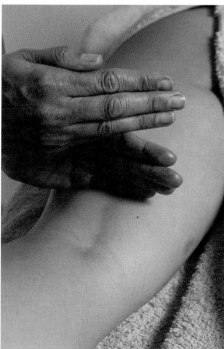

Did you know?

Percutere (the origin of the word percussion) can be broken down into *per* meaning through and *quatere* means to shake. Percussion thus means a shaking through the body.

MASSAGE TECHNIQUES

How to do it

Hacking: hold both hands over the body with palms facing each other and the edge of the little finger closest to the client. The fingers should be together and relaxed and the elbows out, away from the body. Strike the body with alternate hands, with the movement originating from the wrist. As soon as one hand touches the skin let it spring back as the other drops to hack. Begin slowly with a light pressure and build up to a vigorous rhythm with firm pressure. Keep the hands and wrists relaxed to prevent causing pain and keep the rhythm bouncy and light.

Beating: make hands into fists, with the little finger side facing each other. Lower one fist then the other alternately, lifting one fist as the other lowers. Begin slowly with a light pressure and build up to a vigorous rhythm with firm pressure. Keep both hands and wrists relaxed and keep the movement brisk and springy so that the fists bounce away from the body as soon as they touch it and do not thump or cause pain. Pounding should only be used on fleshy areas.

Pounding: Similar to beating except the sides of the fist hit the tissue and the little finger side of the fist faces down towards the clients skin.

Cupping: hold hands out with palm facing up then form 'cup' shapes with the hands. Invert the 'cups' so that the 'inside' is closest to the client's skin. Then, following the same rhythm as hacking, lower one 'cup' then the next alternately. Begin slowly with light pressure and build up to a vigorous rhythm with firm pressure. Keep both hands and wrists relaxed and keep the movement brisk and springy. If done properly, the movement will create a sound similar to the 'clip clop' of horses hooves as air is pushed away from the surface of the skin by the pressure of the cupped hands, thus creating a vacuum.

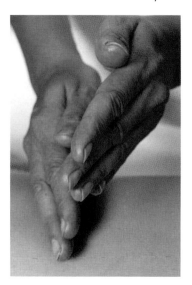

Hacking

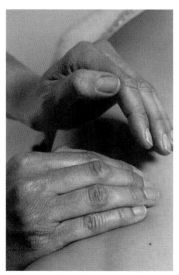

Cupping:

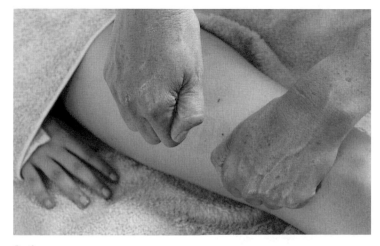

Beating

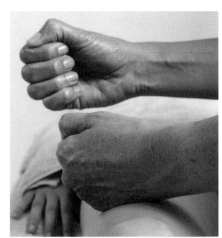

Pounding:

Be careful not to slap.
It is the coming off the body with suction that stimulates the systems of the body, particularly the cardiovascular system. A redness, or erythema, may develop.

Tapotement: this is a very gentle form of percussion, using just the fingertips, which is carried out on delicate or sensitive areas, such as the face. The name derives from *tapoter*, a French word meaning to tap, and tapping is the basis of the technique. Keep the fingers loose and relaxed and tap the area very lightly and gently. Start slowly and build up to a gentle, repetitive and firm rhythm. As with other percussion movements the hands should be relaxed in order to keep the stroke bouncy. This is a soothing movement and should not be heavy or jerky.

When to use it

Percussion should be used as an invigorating, wake-up stroke. If the aim of the whole massage is to stimulate the system rather than soothe it, percussion should form the major part of the treatment. If the aim of the massage is to soothe or relax, percussion can be used towards the end of the treatment, before the final effleurage strokes, to 'wake up' the client's systems. It should not be used on bony or delicate areas.

What does it do?

Percussion is the most invigorating of massage techniques. It improves local and overall circulation, warms the skin and muscles, improves muscle tone both because of the physical effect of the treatment and because of the improved circulation, helps break up fat deposits in fleshy areas and invigorates the nerves.

You now know the classic Swedish massage techniques, how to use them and why. The next section explains other massage techniques.

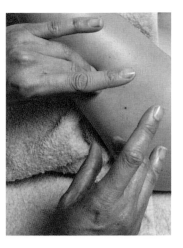
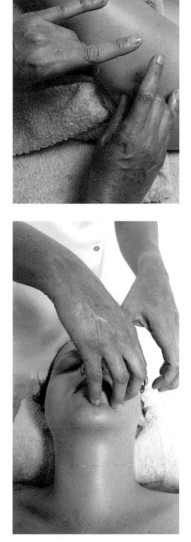
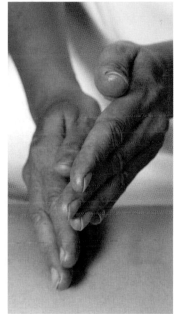
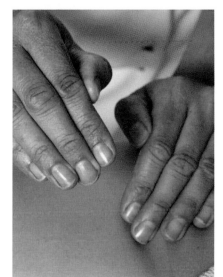

If you remember only one thing...

Percussion is a striking, wake-up stroke. It has a stimulating action on the tissues.

OTHER TECHNIQUES

If you remember only one thing...

Vibration is a pain reliever which clears nerve pathways and helps loosen tightness in the muscles.

What is vibration?

Vibration can be either manual or mechanical. It aims to make the muscle tremble and shake in order to loosen tightness and release tension. Mechanical vibration equipment can be used to produce the same effects.

How to do it

Vibration can be carried out using either one or both hands and either whole palms or just the fingertips. Place the palms of the hands/fingertips on the muscle and, retaining firm, deep contact with the muscle throughout the movement, briskly move the hands/fingertips up and down or from side to side by tensing the arms so much that they shake.

When to use it

When muscles are extremely tight and not responding well to petrissage or frictions.

What does it do?

Vibration helps release pain and tension. It can be a very soothing technique or a very stimulating one, depending on the desired result. It can literally surprise the muscle into releasing its tension.

Passive joint movements

Passive movements require the client to relax and let the therapist gently take a joint (e.g. knee, elbow, shoulder) through its natural range of movement. These movements may help to improve mobility and release tension.

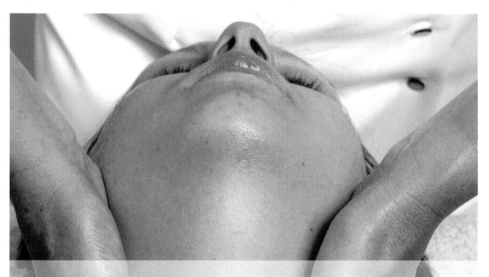

REMEMBER
- Massage movements should always be used with upward pressure towards the heart. This helps venous return and lymphatic drainage.
- During a massage session the therapist should always aim to keep at least one hand in contact with the client, to prevent interrupting the mood of relaxation, and to reassure the client.
- Percussion and petrissage should not be used on bony or delicate areas.
- The therapist should start with light strokes and gentle pressure and build up to deeper strokes and firmer pressure, whilst maintaining a slow rate and rhythm throughout.

GENERAL SUMMARY

Massage techniques and effects

The following is a general summary of the styles of movement or pressure used in massage and their effects on the body. It is intended as a guideline, not an absolute. With some treatments and some clients different effects may result and the techniques may be used differently.

How do I use the techniques in a routine?

The therapist's routine

Per Ling used the following routine: effleurage, petrissage, effleurage, percussion, effleurage. However, all massage therapists will develop their own routines according to the requirements of their clients. The therapist is the source of the massage and thus can control its effects and results. It is the therapist's responsibility to find out about the client's requirements and expectations and plan a routine that will meet them. For example, a client who wants a thorough, invigorating massage will require a routine built around stimulating techniques such as percussion with less focus on relaxing, gentle strokes like effleurage. A client who wants a relaxing massage will require a routine that focuses on effleurage and petrissage with less emphasis on percussion, if it is used at all. Mechanical methods are generally not used in relaxation because they are not as effective as the hands, either for palpating the muscles or for relaxing the client through touch. The time spent on each type of movement and the pressure used will also be determined by the individual's needs and the desired results.

The client's input

Each individual will experience massage techniques differently so that one may find a percussion movement very invigorating whereas another finds it painful. Again the therapist must work with the client to achieve the best results. The aim is to invigorate and/or soothe and at no time should the client's comments, especially with respect to pain, be ignored. The therapist must learn to adapt to each client's pain threshold. Ignoring it will in the short-term prevent the massage from being relaxing and in the long-term may cause damage.

Why are continuous movements necessary?

One hand or both should always be kept on the body during treatment since as soon as the hands are removed the body will register this as the end of the massage and begin to 'change gear', getting ready to dress and leave.

You now know the different techniques used in massage, how and when to perform them and what they do. You also know the importance of the therapist's input and that of the client. The next section explains what a massage medium is and why it is used.

MASSAGE MEDIUMS

What is a massage medium?
A massage medium is a lubricant which helps the therapist's hands to move freely and smoothly over the client's skin. The three most common mediums used are oil, cream and powder.

Massage oils
Oil is the most useful massage medium because it is smooth and light. Massage oils should be of vegetable or plant origin and not too thick or heavy because the heat and pressure of massage movements can make them sticky. Lighter oils, such as grapeseed, are more useful for larger areas because they are smoother. Thicker oils, such as avocado are more useful for smaller areas. Blends of oils can be used either for a blend of properties or to make a more expensive oil go further, e.g. a dense, expensive oil such as evening primrose oil, which is very good for use on dry skin, could be blended with a lighter, less expensive oil such as grapeseed. Mineral oils, such as baby oil, should not be used as they dry the skin.

See Chapter 12 for more information on using oils in aromatherapy massage.

Massage creams
Creams are good for small or delicate areas such as the face or on very dry skin. They tend to be heavier and more oily than oils. As they are absorbed faster than massage oils, they may require more frequent application.

Powder
Powder is useful for oily skin, very hairy clients or on clients who dislike the residues of oils and creams. Swedish massage was traditionally performed using powder because powder prevents the hands from sliding over the surface of the body and allows deeper pressure.

Gels
Gels are normally water based substances, non-oily and usually leave no residue. The majority of massage gels on the market may contain herbal extracts although the formulations may vary from company to company. These gels are useful for clients who prefer to feel less oily, or have naturally oily skins. Gels are often rapidly absorbed and may not be suitable for dry skin types.

Emulsions
The basic component of most cosmetics is an emulsion of oil-in-water, or water-in-oil, in which one component is dispersed as small (0.1μm to 50μm) droplets in the other. The balance chosen will depend on the strength of emollient properties required from a product. The size of the suspended droplets can vary, and the emulsion will become effectively transparent if their diameter is less than about 0.05μm. Most emulsions consist of two components, but it is possible to create more complex emulsions with, for example, water dispersed in the oil phase of an oil-in-water emulsion, to create a water-in-oil-in-water emulsion.

How much medium should I use?
The amount of medium used will depend on the client. In general a full body massage will require about 20-25 ml of oil. Massage of larger clients and those with dry skin will require more medium.

How should massage mediums be stored?
Essential oils are delicate and expensive. It is therefore wise to look after them. They should be stored –
- away from extremes of temperature:

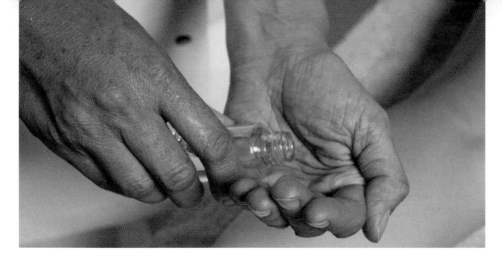

heat will evaporate them and cold can affect their composition

- essential oils should be stored in dark, amber glass bottles (or dark blue glass bottles if kept in the dark or a refrigerator): essential oils are sensitive to ultraviolet light; they should not be stored, or bought, in plastic because it affects the molecular structure of the oil (For more information on essential oils see page 224)
- in tightly sealed bottles: to protect them from evaporating in the air and to stop contact with the air from changing their composition
- out of the reach of children (childproof caps are now available for use with essential oil bottles).
- it is important that carrier/fixed oils are also bottled and stored appropriately, away from air, heat and light. They are susceptible to oxidation and hydrolysis – contamination and degradation by oxygen and water and can turn rancid. Changes in the quality of carrier/fixed oils are usually detectable by changes in colour, odour and viscosity.

How do I apply it?

All massage mediums should first be dispensed into the therapist's hands, rather than straight on to the client's body. This is because the oil, cream or powder will be cold and uncomfortable on the skin if it is not warmed up and evenly distributed. The therapist should

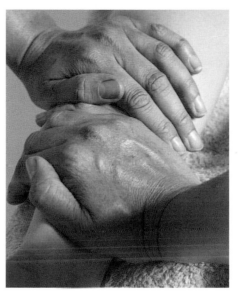

One possible method for applying oil

dispense a small amount into the palm of one hand and then rub the hands together to warm the medium and distribute it smoothly across palms and fingertips. The therapist should then apply the medium using effleurage strokes.

Sensitive skin and allergies

Before using any oil, cream or powder powder, the therapist may wish to carry out a patch test, especially if the client has sensitive skin or allergies. Wash the crook of the elbow with water or water and a mild soap, dry it then rub a small amount of the medium onto the skin. Leave for 24 hours and check for any reactions.

You now know the different techniques and mediums used in massage.

Watch video of this routine on the e-Learning Resource (See page 28)

MASSAGE ROUTINE

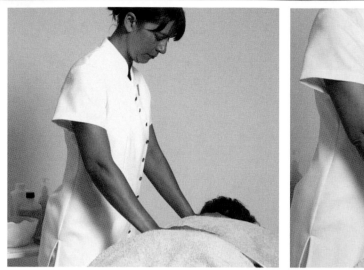

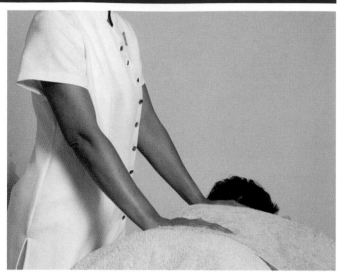

Holding on the back

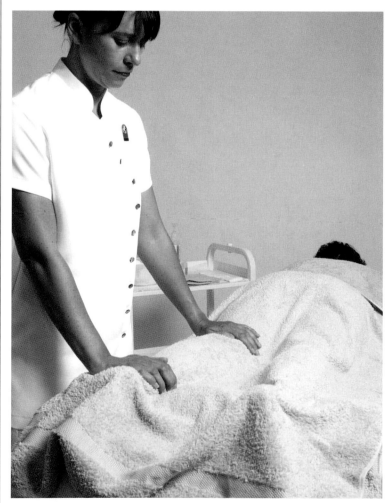

Holding on the feet/ankles

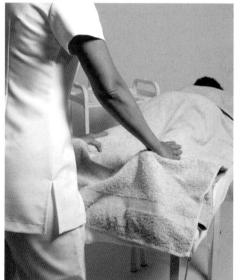

Slowly turn back the towels

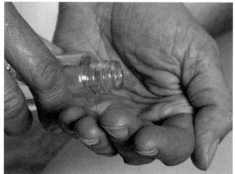

Pouring the oil

MASSAGE

Back of the legs

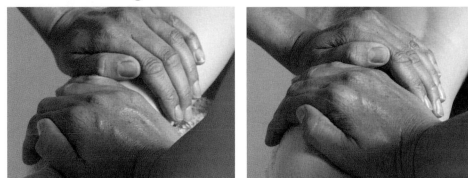

1) Effleurage to spread the oil

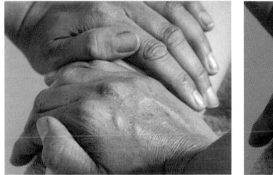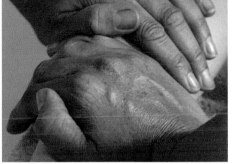

2) Effleurage the whole leg six times

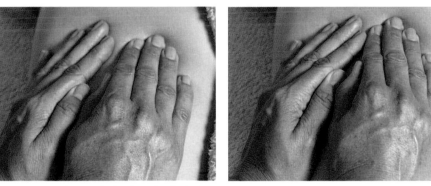

3) Palmar kneading to the back of the thigh six times

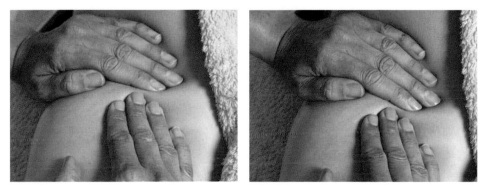

4) Alternate palmar kneading to the back of the thigh six times

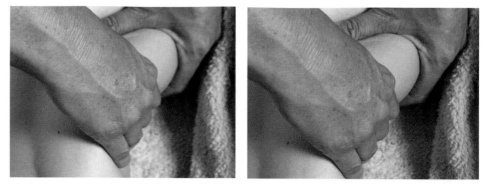

5) Picking up twice all over the back of the thigh.

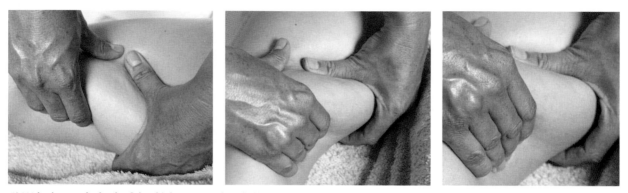

6) Wringing on the back of the thigh to cover the whole area twice

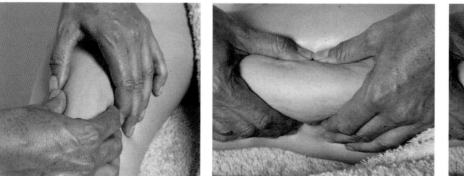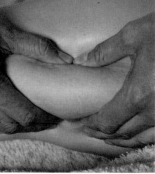

7) Skin rolling on the back of the thigh to cover the whole area twice

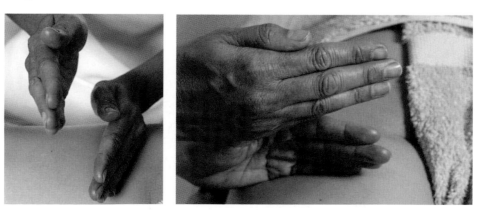

8) Hacking

MASSAGE

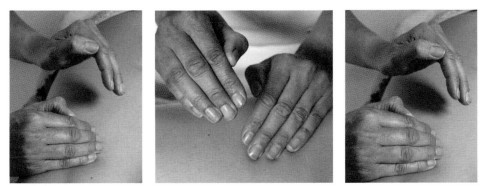

9) Cupping

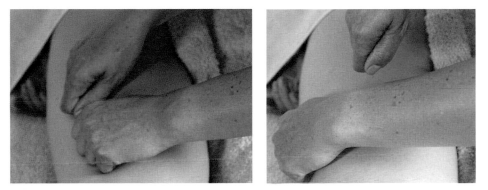

10) Beating

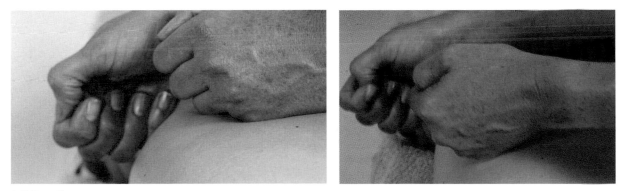

11) Pounding

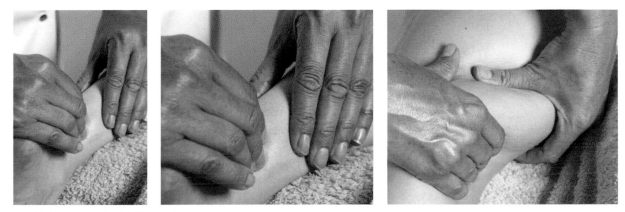

12) Picking up on the Achilles tendon

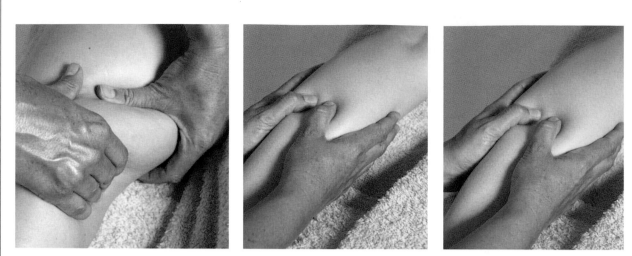

13) *Picking up on the gastrocnemius and soleus twice.*

14) *Split the gastrocnemius three times*

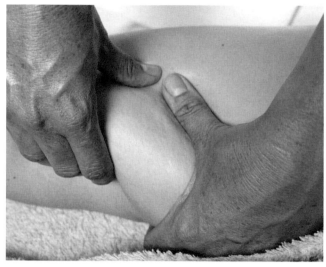

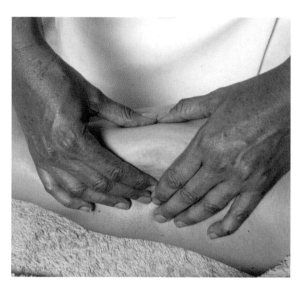

15) *Wringing on the gastroc-nemius and soleus twice*

16) *Skin rolling on the gastrocnemius and soleus twice*

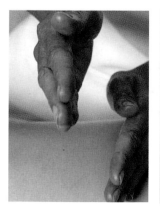

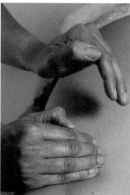

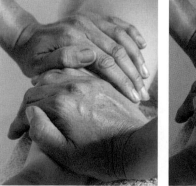

17) *Hacking along the muscle fibres*

18) *Cupping along the muscles fibres*

19) *Effleurage the whole leg six times*

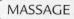

Back *1) Effleurage to spread the oil*

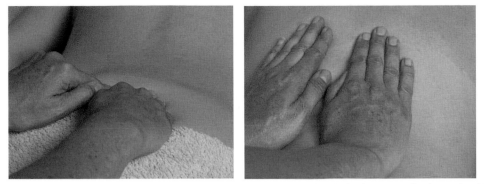

2) Effleurage twice in the middle (either side of the spine), twice slightly further out and twice to the sides of the body

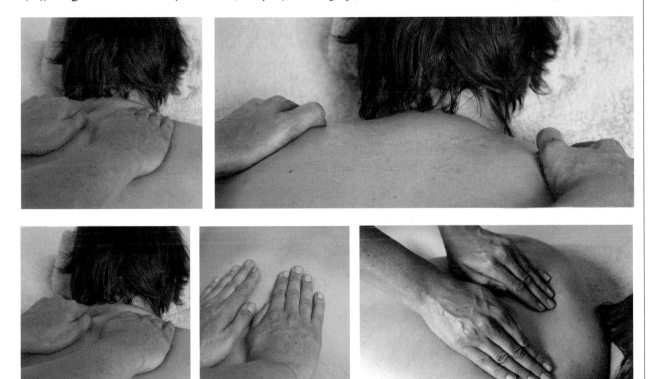

3) Palmar kneading six times in the same pattern

4) Alternate palmar kneading six times in the same pattern

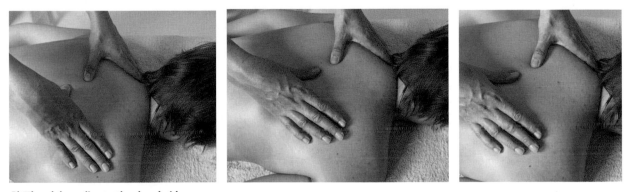

5) Thumb kneading to the rhomboids

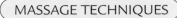

MASSAGE TECHNIQUES

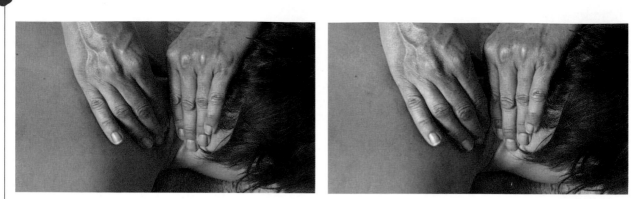

6) Kneading on the neck in the cervical area

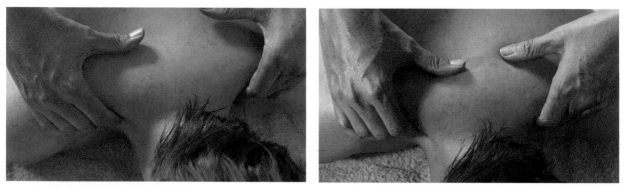

7) Skin rolling on the trapezius three times

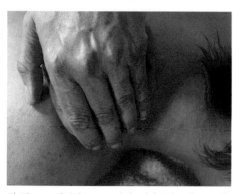 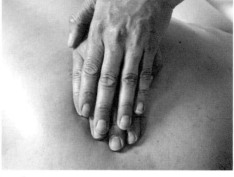

8) Figure of eight around the deltoid and scapula three times

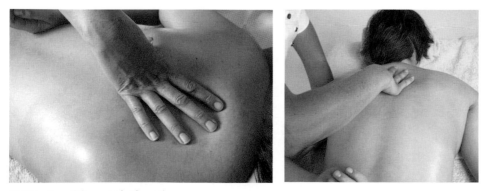

9) Winging of the scapula three times.

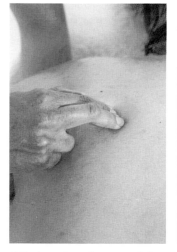 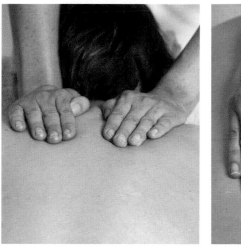 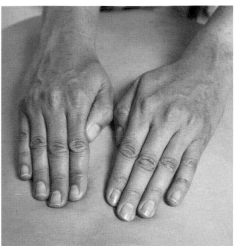

10) *Finger kneading around the scapula three times*

11) *Reverse effleurage six times*

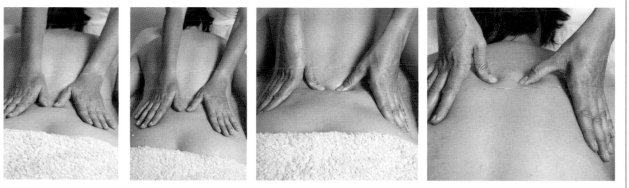

12) *Thumb kneading up either side of the spine three times*

13)   *Thumb kneading the rhomboids three times.*

14)   *Picking up*

15)   *Wringing as before*

16)   *Skin rolling as before*

17)   *Hacking on the hips, upper arms and shoulders*

18)   *Cupping on the hips, upper arms and shoulders*

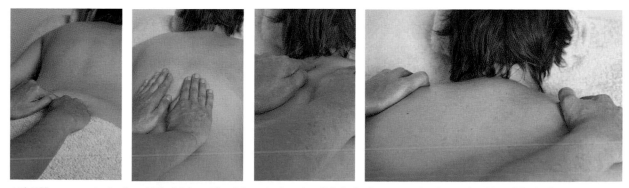

19) *Effleurage twice in the middle (either side of the spine), twice slightly further out and twice to the sides of the body*

Face massage: *Spread the oil over the chest, shoulders, neck and face*

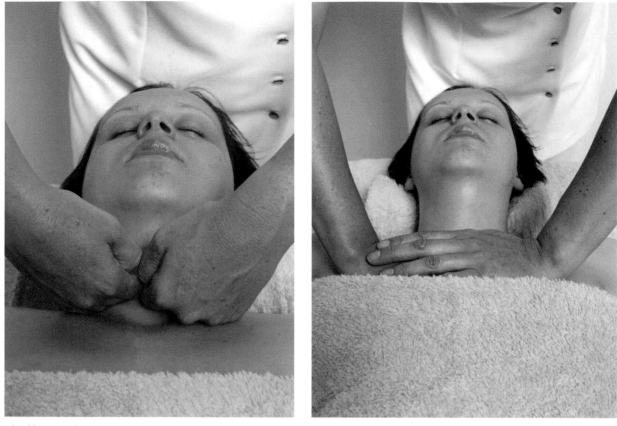

1) Effleurage the neck, chest and shoulders six times, covering the platysma, pectorals, deltoids and trapezius

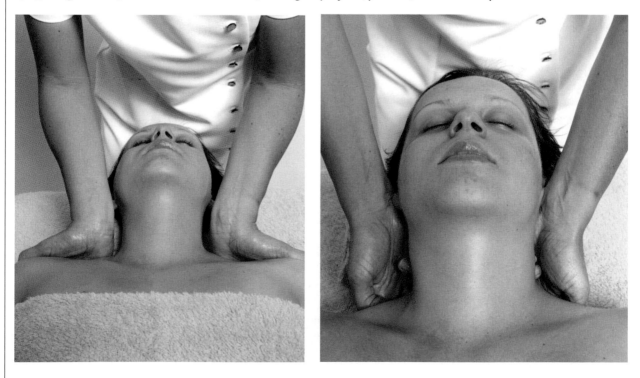

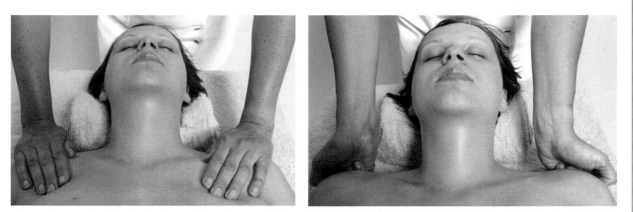

2) Rotations on the deltoids six times with an effleurage in between across the platysma, pectorals and trapezius muscles

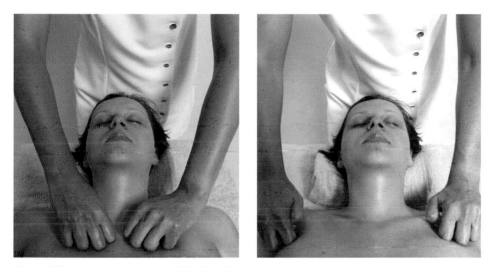

3) Knuckling across the pectorals, deltoids and trapezius six times

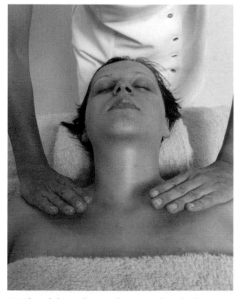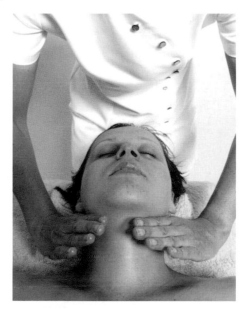

4) Thumb kneading to the trapezius six times

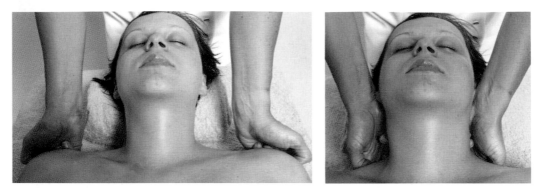

5) Finger kneading along the trapezius into the occipital six times. Turn the client's head slowly to one side

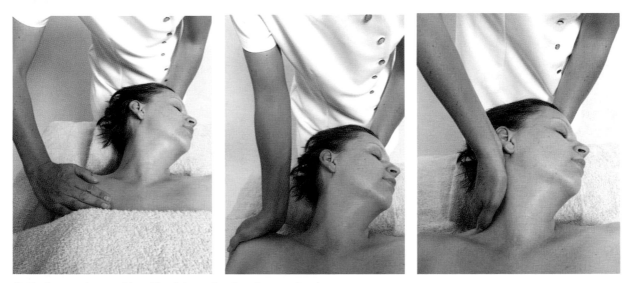

6) Six deep strokes up either side of the neck, using alternate hands,
covering the sternocleido mastoid, the trapezius and platysma muscles

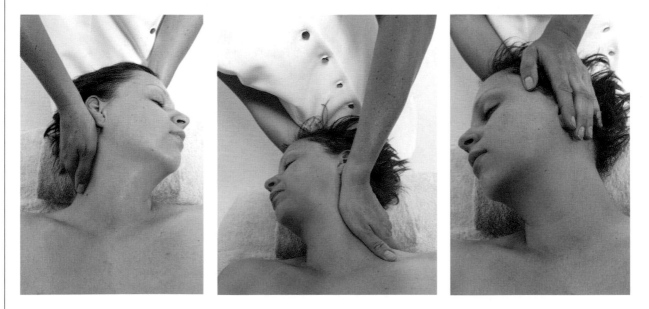

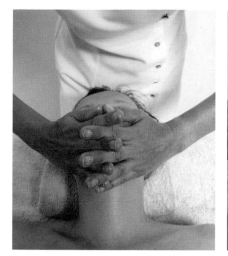
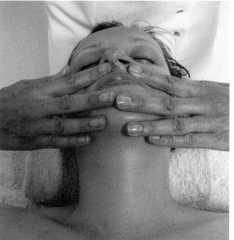
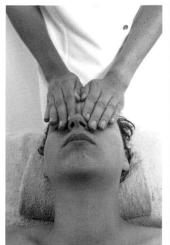

7) *Three full face braces*

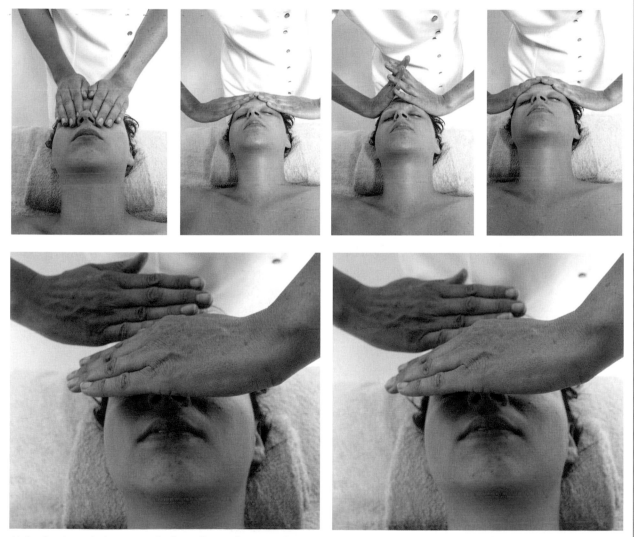

8) *Stroke above the brow over the frontalis muscle twenty times*

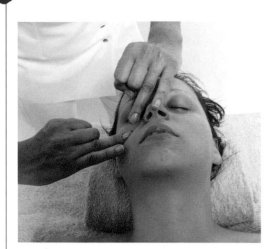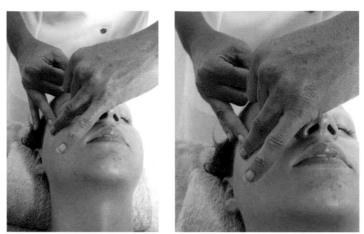

9) Half moon stroking under each eye six times   *10) Alternate stroking at the sides of the eye*

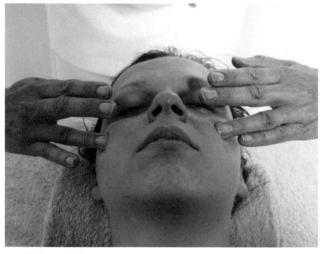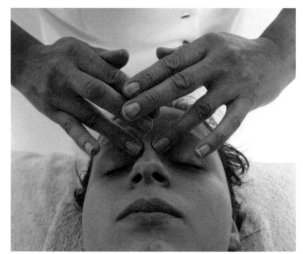

11) Full eye circles

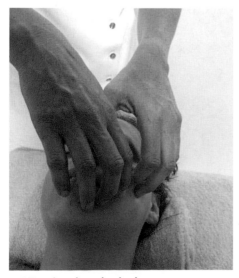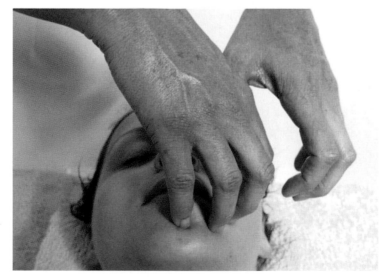

12) Tapping along the cheeks
13) Three full face braces (As stage 7)

14) Glide up to the scalp

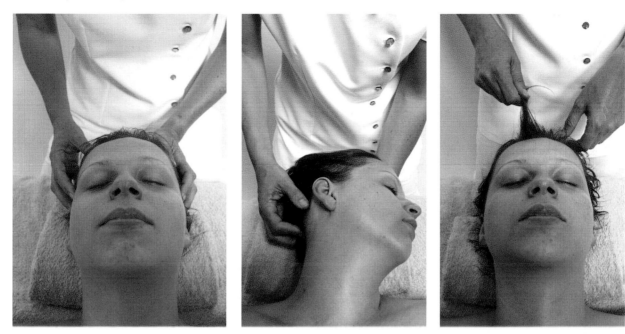

Stroke gently though the hair   *Petrissage*   *Gently pull on the hair*

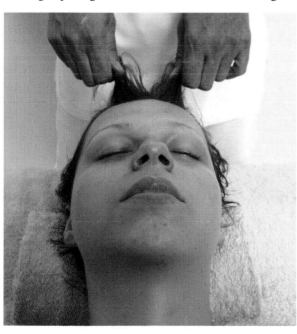
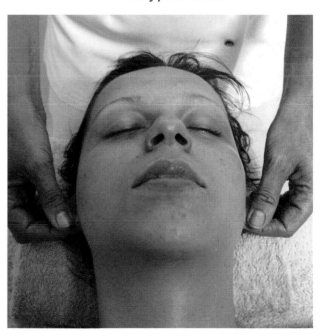

Knead around the edge of the ears

15) Effleurage the neck, chest and shoulders six times (As in stage 1).

16) Rotations on the deltoids six times (Stage 2).

17) Knuckling across the pectorals, deltoids and trapezius six times (Stage 3).

18) Thumb kneading to the trapezius six times (Stage 4)

19) Finger kneading along the trapezius into the occipital six times (Stage 5)

20) Three vibrations into the occipital

MASSAGE TECHNIQUES

Arms   *1) Effleurage to spread the oil.*

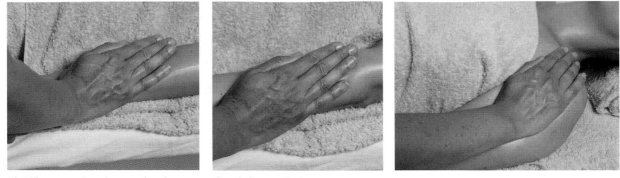

2) Effleurage using alternate hands to cover the whole arm six times

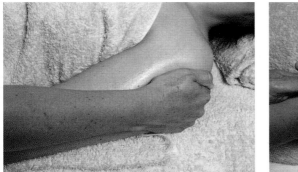
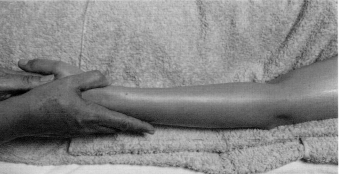

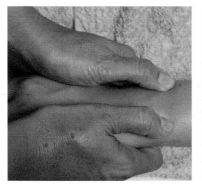
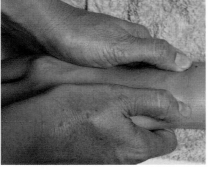
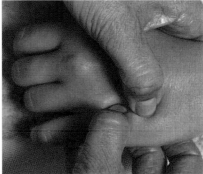

3) Knead around the carpals six times

4) Thumb knead between the metacarpals, little finger to thumb

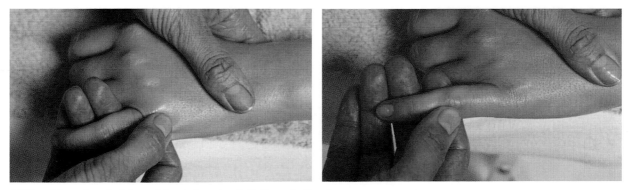

5) Thumb knead on the joints of the phalanges – little finger to thumb

MASSAGE

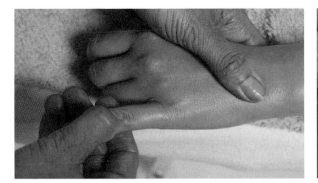
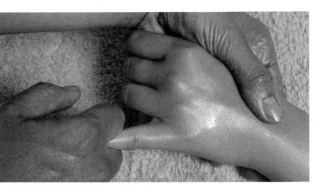

6) *Gentle pulling on the fingers – little finger to thumb*

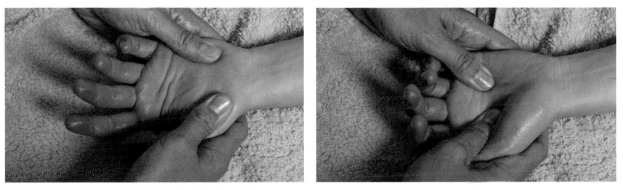

7) *Turn the hand over – thumb knead to thenar and hypothenar eminence*

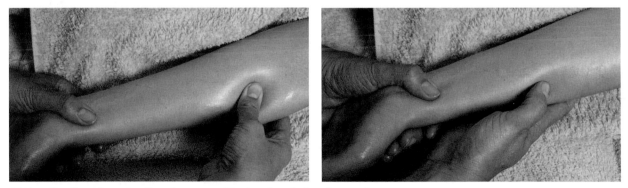

8) *Kneading down from the elbow (superatrochlea lymph nodes) to the carpals*

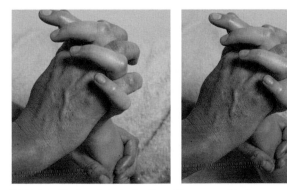
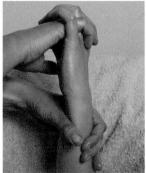
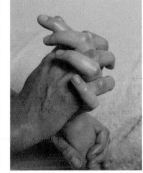

9) *Rotate the hand clockwise three times very slowly*

*Reverse and rotate the hand
anticlockwise three times very slowy*

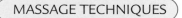
MASSAGE TECHNIQUES

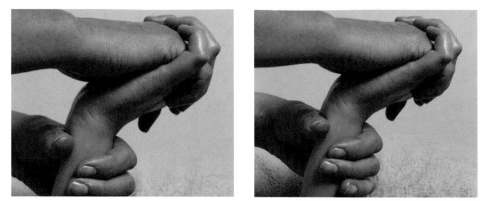

10) Flex and extend the wrist supporting the joint throughout the movement, twice each way

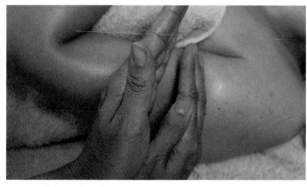
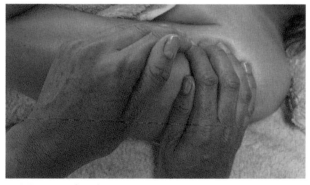

11) Place the client's hand on their opposite shoulder to open up the back of the arm. Palmar knead over the triceps six times

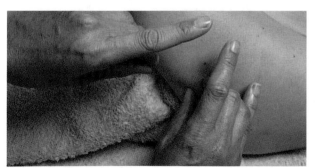
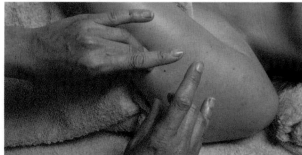

12) Hack over the triceps

13) Cup over the triceps

14) Pincement on the triceps

Effleurage using alternate hands to cover the whole arm six times (As in 2).

MASSAGE

Abdomen

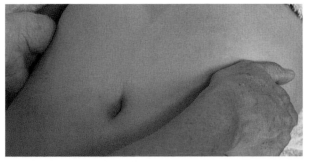
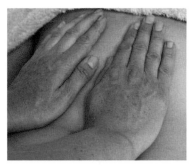

1) Effleurage to spread the oil

2) Effleurage six times, two to the centre, two moving out and two to the sides of the abdominal region

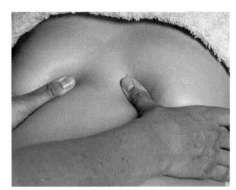
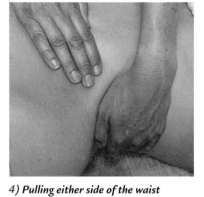
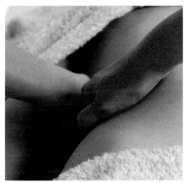

3) Six breathing movements

4) Pulling either side of the waist

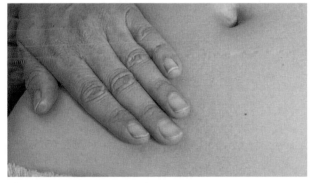
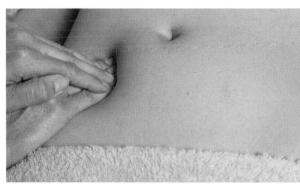

5) Circular effleurage, around the colon

6) Reinforced kneading around the colon

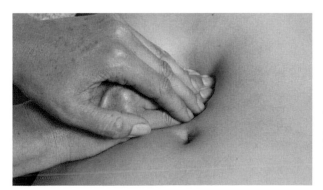
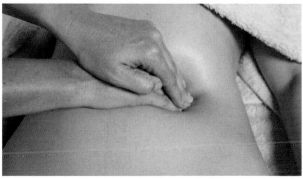

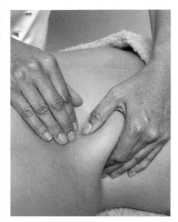
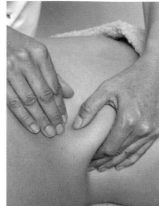
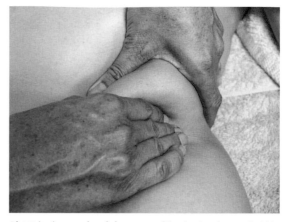

7) Picking up on the abdomen working in the shape of a W

8) Wringing on the abdomen working in the shape of a W

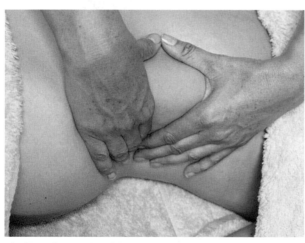
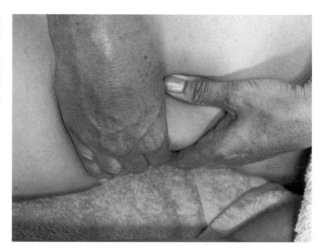

9) Skin rolling on the abdomen working in the shape of a W

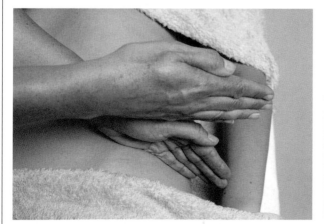
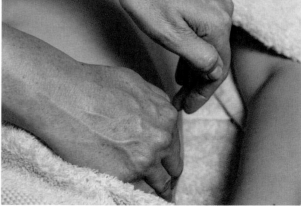

10) Hacking to the hips

11) Cupping on the hips

12) Effleurage six times, two to the centre, two moving out and two to the sides of the abdominal region (As in point 2).

13) Finish with deep pressure in the small of the back

MASSAGE

Front of legs

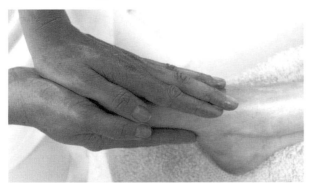

1) Effleurage to spread the oil

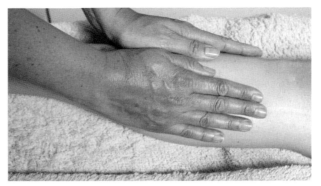

2) Effleurage the whole leg six times

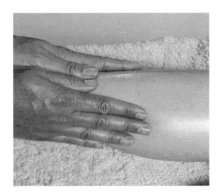

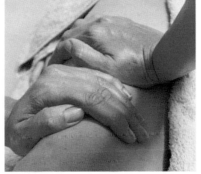

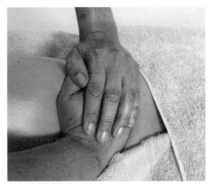

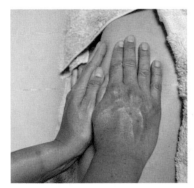

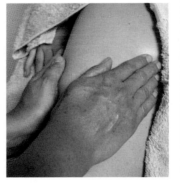

3) Palmar kneading to the top of the thigh six times

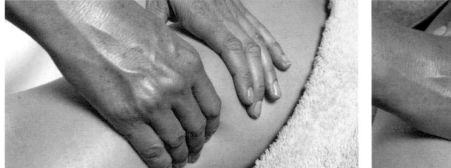

4) Alternate palmar kneading to the top of the thigh six times

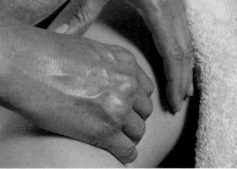

5) Picking up twice on the front of the thigh

MASSAGE TECHNIQUES

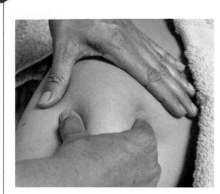
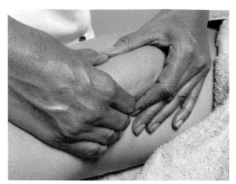
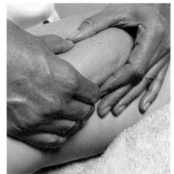

6) Wringing on the front of the thigh twice

7) Skin rolling on the front of the thigh twice

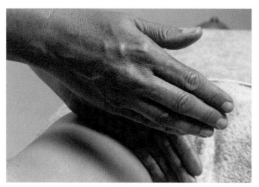
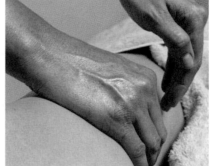
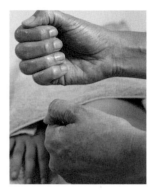

8) Hacking

9) Cupping

10) Beating

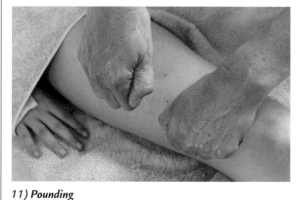
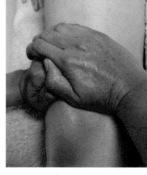
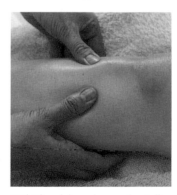

11) Pounding

12) Effleurage up to and including patella six times

13) Thumb knead around patella three times

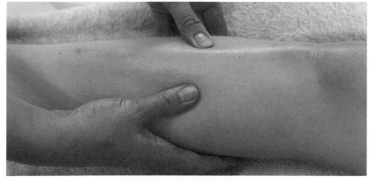
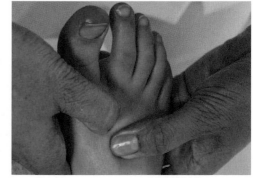

14) Knead either side of the tibia twice moving down to the tarsals

15) Thumb knead between the metatarsals, little toe to big toe

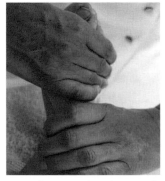 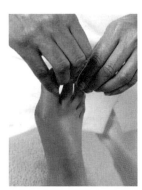 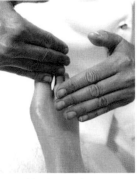 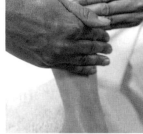

16) Full toe rotations (once each way, all the toes together)

17) Picking on the toes

18) Whipping on the toes

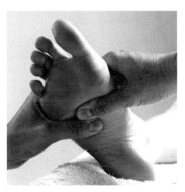 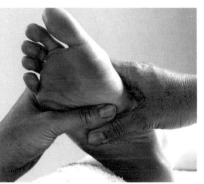 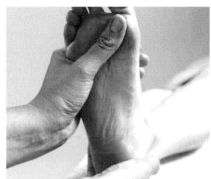

19) Cross frictions down the foot using the thumbs, then working back up

20) Flex and extend the foot, twice each way

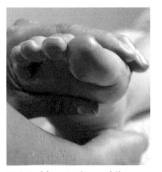 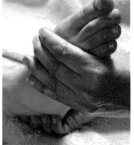

21) Ankle rotations whilst supporting the ankle joint, three times one way then reverse

22) Effleurage the whole leg six times (As in point 2)

Cover the leg gently with the towel.
Hold onto the client's feet through the towels.
Energise with the palms of your hands on the client's feet
Move up the couch and place one hand on the client's abdomen on top of the towels and the other on the client's forehead
Then take your hands away from the client so slowly that they feel as though you are still touching them.

MASSAGE TECHNIQUES

CASE STUDY - CLIENT PROFILE

Mrs MB is 42 years old. She is married and has no children although she is stepmother to 4 grown up children.

She lives with her husband who is an engineer. She is employed full time as a Management Accountant. Her office is based a short distance from her home so she is able to walk to work most days, depending on the weather.

Last year was stressful for her – she was made redundant from a job that she really enjoyed. However, she was quickly re-employed within a month, but she had some misgivings about her new job. Compared to previous jobs she felt under-utilised and this became a source of frustration for her. Consequently, after only four months she resigned. Due to the high demand for her skills, she found a new job and started at a new company within less than a month.

In the middle of all of the job moves, she got married – organising the wedding completely by herself within a short space of time. This added to her stress levels although she appeared to cope well with all the additional planning necessary. She has a very busy life both socially and professionally. She rates her stress levels as low – work 4/10 and home 2/10 and she has a positive, pro-active approach to life. Mrs MB is a keen amateur triathlete who had a regular training schedule. However, before her last event she developed severe back pain that resulted in a visit to a physiotherapist. She had to withdraw from her last two races, a triathlon and half-marathon and has now stopped her training programme completely. She did not visit her doctor, but the physiotherapist recommended remedial exercises that have helped. She has recently started to exercise again, swimming once a week and cycling occasionally but not at the same level as previously practised.

She suffers no contraindications and is generally in very good health. She eats a healthy diet, mostly organic and is a non-smoker. She does suffer with occasional eczema on her hands and her skin is slightly dry but she feels that this is age related.

Mrs MB feels that her back problems may be due to over training, particularly increased running and the change in her office environment. She thinks that massage may help to improve her circulation and relax her back muscles and prevent aches and pains.

She has signed an informed consent form, and has been made fully aware of the treatment and its effects.

Reason for treatment

Intermittent back ache/pain/stiffness – back pain started in August due to an increased running programme and a change in work/office environment. It has now eased but Mrs MB is anxious that it may return.

Treatment Plan

A full body massage once a week for four weeks is proposed using the full range of classical massage movements with particular emphasis on the lower back/problem area to help prevent muscle stiffness.

Client Consultation Form – Holistic

College Name:
College Number:
Student Name:
Student Number:
Date: 05/11

Client Name: Mrs MB
Address: Derby

Profession: Management Accountant
Tel. No: Day
                Eve

PERSONAL DETAILS

Age group: ❏ Under 20   ❏ 20–30   ❏ 30–40   ☑ 40–50   ❏ 50–60   ❏ 60+

Lifestyle: ☑ Active   ❏ Sedentary   Regular exercise undertaken and she usually walks to work

Last visit to the doctor: ❏ Jan   Consulted a local physiotherapist about back pain when it occurred. Did not visit

GP Address: Derby   the doctor as she felt that a physiotherapist would offer more help.

No. of children (if applicable): 0

Date of last period (if applicable): 29/10

CONTRAINDICATIONS REQUIRING MEDICAL PERMISSION – in circumstances where medical permission cannot be obtained clients must give their informed consent in writing prior to treatment (select where/if appropriate):

❏ Pregnancy
❏ Cardiovascular conditions (thrombosis, phlebitis, hypertension, hypotension, heart conditions)
❏ Haemophilia
❏ Any condition already being treated by a GP or another complementary practitioner
❏ Medical oedema
❏ Osteoporosis
❏ Arthritis
❏ Nervous/Psychotic conditions
❏ Epilepsy
❏ Recent operations
❏ Any dysfunction of the nervous system (e.g. Multiple sclerosis, Parkinson's disease, Motor neurone disease)

❏ Bell's Palsy
❏ Trapped/Pinched nerve (e.g. sciatica)
❏ Inflamed nerve
❏ Cancer
❏ Postural deformities
❏ Spastic conditions
❏ Kidney infections
❏ Whiplash
❏ Slipped disc
☑ Undiagnosed pain
❏ When taking prescribed medication
❏ Acute rheumatism
❏ Asthma
❏ Diabetes

Mrs MB is not suffering any contraindications that require medical permission but has experienced intermittent back pain. The treatment has been fully explained and she has signed an informed consent form.

CONTRAINDICTIONS THAT RESTRICT TREATMENT (select where/if appropriate):

❏ Fever
❏ Contagious or infectious diseases
❏ Under the influence of recreational drugs or alcohol
❏ Diarrhoea and vomiting
❏ Skin diseases
❏ Undiagnosed lumps and bumps
❏ Localised swelling
❏ Inflammation
❏ Varicose veins
❏ Pregnancy (abdomen)
❏ Cuts
❏ Bruises

❏ Abrasions
❏ Scar tissues (2 years for major operation and 6 months for a small scar)
❏ Sunburn
❏ Hormonal implants
❏ Cervical spondylitis
❏ Gastric ulcers
❏ Abdomen (first few days of menstruation depending how the client feels)
❏ Haematoma
❏ Hernia
❏ Recent fractures (minimum 3 months)

WRITTEN PERMISSION REQUIRED BY:

❏ GP/Specialist   ☑ Informed consent
Either of which should be attached to the consultation form.

66

PERSONAL INFORMATION (select if/where appropriate):

Muscular/Skeletal problems: ☑ Back ☐ Aches/Pain ☐ Stiff joints ☐ Headaches

Client experiences intermittent back stiffness. She consulted a physiotherapist to help her deal with a problem resulting from over training in August.

Digestive problems: ☐ Constipation ☑ Bloating ☐ Liver/Gall bladder ☐ Stomach

Client suffers bloating associated with menstruation occasionally Circulation: Heart

Circulation: ☐ Heart ☐ Blood pressure ☐ Fluid retention ☐ Tired legs ☐ Varicose veins
☑ Cellulite ☐ Kidney problems ☐ Cold hands and feet ☐ Borderline low blood pressure 110/80

Client has light cellulite deposits on thighs. Therapist observations note that the client has very toned thighs but poor circulation in the area.

Gynaecological: ☐ Irregular periods ☐ P.M.T ☐ Menopause ☐ H.R.T ☐ Pill ☐ Coil

Nervous system: ☐ Migraine ☐ Tension ☐ Stress ☐ Depression

Immune system: ☐ Prone to infections ☐ Sore throats ☐ Colds ☐ Chest ☐ Sinuses

Regular antibiotic/medication taken? ☐ Yes ☑ No

If yes, which ones:

Herbal remedies taken? ☐ Yes ☑ No

If yes, which ones:

Ability to relax: ☐ Good ☑ Moderate ☐ Poor

Sleep patterns: ☑ Good ☐ Poor ☐ Average No. of hours 8

Do you see natural daylight in your workplace? ☑ Yes ☐ No

Do you work at a computer? ☑ Yes ☐ No If yes how many hours 1

Do you eat regular meals? ☑ Yes ☐ No

Do you eat in a hurry? ☑ Yes ☐ No

Do you take any food/vitamin supplements? ☐ Yes ☑ No

If yes, which ones:

How many portions of each of these items does your diet contain per day?

Fresh fruit: 1 Fresh vegetables: 4 Protein: 2 source? *Meat, fish, cheese*

Dairy produce: 0 Sweet things: 1 Added salt: 0 Added sugar: 0

How many units of these drinks do you consume per day?

Tea: 0 Coffee: 6 Fruit juice: 1 Water: 0 Soft drinks: 0 Others: 1

Do you suffer from food allergies? ☐ Yes ☑ No Bingeing? ☐ Yes ☑ No

Overeating? ☐ Yes ☑ No *Mrs GH is unsure is sinus problems are due to food or other allergy*

Do you smoke? ☑ No ☐ Yes How many per day?

Do you drink alcohol? ☐ No ☑ Yes How many units per day? *1 Has a glass of red wine in the evening*

Do you exercise? ☐ None ☐ Occasional ☐ Irregular ☑ Regular

Types: *Usually walking, running, cycling as part of an ongoing regime. Currently not exercising due to back stiffness/pain*

What is your skin type? ☑ Dry ☐ Oil ☐ Combination ☐ Sensitive ☐ Dehydrated *Client feels that skin is becoming drier with age. She does not take any oil based supplements such as evening primrose oil.*

Do you suffer/have you suffered from: ☐ Dermatitis ☐ Acne ☑ Eczema ☐ Psoriasis
☐ Allergies ☐ Hay Fever ☐ Asthma ☐ Skin cancer

Client suffers mild eczema on her hands occasionally

Stress level: 1–10 (10 being the highest)

At work 4   At home 2

Client rates her stress levels as low for both work and home.

She has a very positive approach to life generally.

TREATMENT 1 - 05/11

Details of how the therapist conducted the treatment

The room was a little cold so additional heating was necessary to ensure client comfort. A full body massage was performed, with extra work/emphasis on the lower back, lumbar, sacral and gluteal regions. The massage medium chosen was grapeseed oil which is light and easily absorbed. Although the client does not suffer a nut allergy, she has a strong dislike of nuts and nut products so I felt it unwise to use sweet almond oil. It was necessary to adjust the pressure used on the back as the client was quite sensitive – experiencing mild discomfort during petrissage on the sacral area. I used a lighter pressure for these movements that the client could tolerate.

Details of how the client felt during and after the treatment

Mrs MB had come straight from work so she was very alert. She had experienced massage before so was not apprehensive about the treatment. However, as this was her first treatment with a different therapist, she talked throughout the treatment and was very interested in the different techniques experienced. No additional support was required by the client. Some discomfort was felt in the sacral area, so pressure was applied within the client's tolerance to help with

relaxation. She felt relaxed and refreshed after the treatment, not sleepy and said that her back felt looser.

Details of homecare advice given

I sat Mrs MB up slowly and she was given a glass of water immediately after the massage to help flush out any accumulated toxins. She was advised to increase her water intake as she currently drinks no water in addition to her daily coffee, herbal tea and fruit juice. She could also try to cut down on her caffeine intake. She was given exercises to perform by her physiotherapist to improve the flexibility in her back so it is important that she continues with these daily. She was also advised to go home and relax for the rest of the evening if possible.

Reflective practice

At the end of the first treatment I felt pleased with the outcome. I did feel that Mrs MB would have benefited from the treatment more if she had remained quiet throughout rather than talking, but this seems to be quite common for clients during their first few sessions. It is important to build a rapport with the client and many find it stress-relieving. It is also a good way of noting things that they might have forgotten to mention during the consultation. I need to work out a way to ask clients to be quiet in a polite way!

TREATMENT 2 - 12/11

Details of how the therapist conducted the treatment

Although Mrs MB felt 'looser' after the last massage, the back stiffness returned quite quickly – within the next day. However, she felt that she slept better after the treatment. There have been no changes to Mrs MB's overall health this week.

A full body massage was performed, again with emphasis on the lower back/sacral area, using a full range of massage movements.
Although Mrs MB stated that she had cellulite on her legs during the initial consultation, I found that her legs were very well toned. As a result I needed to

apply more pressure in order to work the tissues adequately, particularly with the wringing and finger rolling movements. The skin did feel quite cold to the touch in these areas though, perhaps indicating poor circulation.

Details of how the client felt during and after the treatment

Mrs MB arrived straight from work feeling slightly harassed. She then announced that she was on a tight deadline and had to leave in just over one hour. She appeared quite tense throughout the massage and it was obvious that her mind was buzzing with thoughts of the rest of the evening. Whilst she may have experienced some of the physical benefits of massage, such as increased circulation, I was sure that the psychological effects this evening were poor as she seemed quite alert throughout the treatment.
She experienced less discomfort this week in the lumbar/sacral area, so I
was able to apply a little more pressure and work for longer. I still avoided the use of the tapotement movements on the gluteal region.

I sat her up slowly, even though she needed to get going quickly. She said that she felt relaxed and comfortable but after her glass of water, she dressed and left quickly.

Details of homecare advice given

Mrs MB was again advised to increase her water intake. She has been trying this week but kept forgetting. I suggested that she keep a bottle of water on her desk or have a glass of water each time she has a cup of coffee. She is continuing with the physiotherapist recommended exercises. The next treatment will be in one week.

Reflective practice

I felt I rushed through the routine and I forgot some movements. I performed the massage too quickly as I was conscious throughout of the client's time limits. I completed the whole routine in approximately 50 minutes rather than just over an hour. She did not relax fully but appeared to enjoy the treatment nevertheless. I felt disappointed that I let the client's mood affect my performance and I need to be conscious of this for each client.

TREATMENT 3 - 19/11

Details of how the therapist conducted the treatment

Mrs MB has had a very busy week, frequently staying at work much later than planned. Again she seems quite tense, but is looking forward to the treatment. Her lower back stiffness eased slightly this week but because she has been busy, she has only managed one of her recommended exercises each day. She thinks the stiffness is due to increased time at her desk, looking at a computer. However, she has altered her desk layout to prevent back strain/stretching incorrectly to reach files etc. She feels more relaxed mentally. Full body massage utilising complete range of

massage movements. Client experienced discomfort/stiffness in right shoulder and upper trapezius – right hand side, so light petrissage movements were performed, checking the client's tolerance. Her skin absorbed the oil well. Hyperaemia was evident particularly on the edge of the scapula/rhomboid region – right hand side. I was able to work over the lumbar/sacral area more fully this week without Mrs MB experiencing any discomfort.

Details of how the client felt during and after the treatment

She felt a little tense and tired due to her

increased workload but was looking forward to relaxing. She was not really conscious of the tension in her upper back muscles until I worked over them (rhomboids, trapezius), when they became quite painful to touch. Her forearms were also tense and tender when I performed petrissage movements draining to the supratrochlear lymph nodes. She has spent many hours this week inputting data on her computer, sitting in the same position for a long time. She was very quiet this week and appeared to relax fully. She felt completely relaxed at the end of the treatment.

Details of homecare advice given

A glass of water was given to Mrs MB immediately after treatment. She has managed to increase her water intake this week and will try to maintain it this week. However, her busy week has meant that she has not performed as many of her exercises, only managing one every morning. She is keen to start her training regime again shortly so we discussed the importance of warming up and cooling down exercises. She admits that whilst she

is aware of the correct techniques, she does not always use them fully. She is pleased with the effects of regular massage and will continue with it and increasing her back exercises to maintain and improve flexibility. Her new desk layout should also help ease her back strain, as she now has everything within easy reach. Decaffeinated coffee is now available in her office and she is trying to alternate it with normal coffee to cut down her caffeine intake.

Reflective practice

I felt more confident with the routine this evening. It also helped that tonight Mrs MB seemed more relaxed from the start. She did not chat to me so I was able to concentrate fully and felt that the massage was more beneficial as a result. Last week the treatment outcome was affected as Mrs MB was unable to relax afterwards. The immediate effects of the treatment were short lived as she was forced to rush to another appointment immediately after. Treatment scheduling is important as relaxation time after a session is advisable.

TREATMENT 4 - 26/11

Details of how the therapist conducted the treatment

Mrs MB arrived for her treatment in a cheerful and relaxed manner. Her workload is still higher than normal but at the weekend she completed a long bicycle ride with no ill effects afterwards. Although she is currently working longer hours she feels calm and able to cope with the demands of her job. Her back stiffness seems to be easing and her workspace reorganisation seems to be making things easier as she is no longer stretching awkwardly to reach files and documentation that she needs. Full body massage using complete range

of massage movements. Frictions used on the rhomboids and trapezius, again erythema evident particularly on the right hand side. However, this was not as uncomfortable as last week and her shoulder feels less stiff. Knots in the rhomboid area were not as firm this week but petrissage was used to improve the circulation, break down fibrous build up and eliminate lactic acid from tension. The lumbar/sacral area was less tense, although some of this tension appears to have transferred to the upper back but I can now work this area fully without discomfort to the client.

Details of how the client felt during and after the treatment

Although her work-load has increased due to the time of year, she feels happy and able to cope in her new job. Has found weekly treatments very beneficial and they have encouraged her to make some other simple changes which are helping with back tension. The back massage was more comfortable this week, and the trapezius/shoulder area less painful. This seems to be more of a problem than the lower back now, but may ease as her workload normalises shortly. Care was still taken during the back massage with regard to sensitive areas but Mrs MB fully receptive to all massage movements performed firmly on the rest of the body. She feels that the effects of the treatment have been cumulative and she feels relaxed for longer between sessions.

Details of homecare advice given

Mrs MB was given a glass of water immediately after the treatment. She is continuing to drink more water and reduce her caffeine intake – she has graduated onto fully decaffeinated this week. If she is starting to increase her exercise levels and feels stiff as a result she could take a warm bath in the evenings to relax the muscles before bed. She must also ensure that she warms up/cools down before and after exercise as she begins to build up her fitness levels again. Massage treatments are recommended at least once per month or as required as a preventative measure and to continue relaxation. She should also continue to perform the exercises recommended by her physiotherapist as they seem to be helping prevent stiffness, even though she is only managing to perform a limited amount daily.

Reflective Practice

It was very interesting to observe the effects of an increased workload/change in work patterns on her posture/muscles. This had a direct effect on my massage routine and the emphasis in a treatment. I was able to identify tight muscles/problem areas even though she did not necessarily point them out to me. I then adjusted my treatment and spent more time working on these areas to release the tension and increase the blood flow. It was also a good experience working on a client with specific needs i.e. relief from pain/muscular tension. It was much easier to note improvements than if working on someone who just wants general relaxation. The pain/discomfort here could be used as a guide to treatment effectiveness/success. It was interesting to see how the client's mood affected my treatments – particularly in terms of speed. When the client was stressed and anxious about time, I allowed myself to be influenced instead of focusing on making the client relax through a deep and slow massage. It was helpful to work with someone who was clearly interested in helping herself regain fitness, flexibility and prevent further pain or injury. I look forward to continuing to work with this client throughout her return to fitness and forthcoming competitions.

OVERALL CONCLUSION

Mrs MB has benefited from weekly massages, coping with a heavy workload and using the treatment sessions to unwind. She has become more aware of her posture and has changed her desk around to prevent further damage and feels that this is helping. She is more alert during the day and feels that drinking more water has helped. She will continue to drink decaffeinated coffee at work. Mrs MB is fit and body aware, but she must be careful not to over exert herself as she tries to regain her fitness levels. She has found that the massages have made her more aware of how she is feeling physically and hopes that this will guide and help her not to overdo her training when she starts properly. Not all clients undertake home/aftercare advice. It was very interesting to see how improvements in health could be made when the client takes advice and makes changes.

50% OFF!
FULL ACCESS

DON'T FORGET NOW YOU CAN USE A RANGE OF ONLINE LEARNING RESOURCES FOR JUST £10 (NORMAL RRP £20)

The Massage e-Learning Resource has been designed to enhance your learning experience

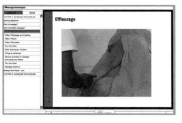

☐ Bring knowledge to life with videos of each technique as well as a full massage routine

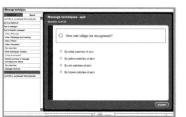

☐ Manage your learning with step-by-step modules and integrated 'classroom' sessions

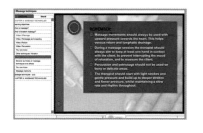

☐ Absorb information on key topics with interactive exercises and learning activities

To login to use these **e-learning resources**, visit **www.emspublishing.co.uk/massage** and follow the onscreen instructions

AN INTRODUCTORY GUIDE TO

Massage

4 Effects and benefits of massage

In Brief

Massage has an immediate physiological effect on the local area of the body being worked on and it also affects the whole body through stimulation and relaxation of the muscles and the nerves. It has physiological and psychological benefits and can affect all the body systems in a positive way.

Learning objectives

The target knowledge of this chapter is:
- physiological effects and benefits of massage
- psychological effects and benefits of massage
- effects of massage on different body systems.

THE EFFECTS AND BENEFITS OF MASSAGE

What are the effects of massage?

The effects of massage are twofold: physiological (relating to the physical structure of the body) and psychological (relating to the mind). When the body is massaged, the mechanics (i.e. the physical action of manipulating tissue) affect the local area of the massage, whereas the nervous stimulation (i.e. the response of the nerves to touch and movement), affects the whole body. Evidently the positive benefits of massage for the physical body will affect the psychological body and vice-versa. However, for the purposes of study they have been divided into physiological and psychological.

Physiological

In the short term massage will:

- improve skin tone and colour by removing dead cells (desquamating) and improving circulation
- encourage better circulation therefore more efficient delivery of nutrients and oxygen to cells and more efficient waste removal
- encourage deeper and therefore more efficient and relaxed breathing

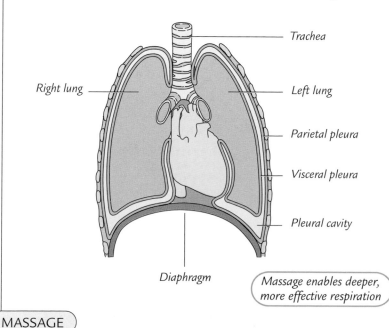

- Trachea
- Right lung
- Left lung
- Parietal pleura
- Visceral pleura
- Pleural cavity
- Diaphragm

Massage enables deeper, more effective respiration

- encourage better lymph drainage and reduce swelling
- relieve muscle fatigue, soreness and stiffness
- relieve tired, stiff joints
- promote general relaxation
- sedate or stimulate the nervous system (depending on type of massage performed)
- encourage sleep
- speed up digestion and waste removal.

In the long term massage will:

- improve skin elasticity
- improve circulation
- boost immunity
- improve muscle suppleness
- improve neural communication and relax the nervous system (preventing, for example, muscle spasms caused by anxiety)
- enable deeper, more effective respiration
- relieve insomnia
- balance the digestive system
- lower high blood pressure.

Psychological

In the short term massage will:

- relax the body, thereby reducing tension and the effects of stress
- relax the mind, thereby reducing anxiety and its effects
- soothe and comfort the client
- give a 'lift' to the emotions and increase positive feelings
- increase energy by invigorating all body systems and reducing fatigue.

In the long term massage will:

- enable sustained relaxation of body and mind
- improve body image, awareness and general self-esteem
- increase energy levels as less energy is spent in holding the body in a state of tension and strain (both physical and mental).

THE SYSTEMS OF THE BODY

The first part of this section explains the effects of massage on the systems that are directly affected. The second part explains the effects on systems that benefit more indirectly.

The cell

Although when a massage is carried out it is not necessary to think of every cell and the effects on it, it helps to recognise that what happens on a global level in a massage also happens at a cellular level. Since massage improves the workings of, and invigorates, body systems, it has the same effect at a cellular level. The delivery of nutrients, oxygen and water, and the removal of carbon dioxide, toxins and waste is faster and more efficient, digestion and respiration are improved and each cell can therefore work at its optimum level.

The skin

The skin is the most obvious part of the body to benefit from massage. The therapist is in constant contact with it throughout the duration of the massage and this not only invigorates the skin but also soothes and relaxes the client.

The effects of massage include:

- **improved skin colour:** poor skin colour is often associated with poor circulation; massage boosts the circulation and thus invigorates skin colour;
- **improved skin tone and texture:** the constant stroking and rubbing of the skin helps speed up desquamation (the removal of dead skin cells) and this encourages the regeneration of the skin cells and better tone;
- **improved elasticity:** massage encourages the production of sebum, the skin's natural oil, which helps keep the skin lubricated and prevents dryness.

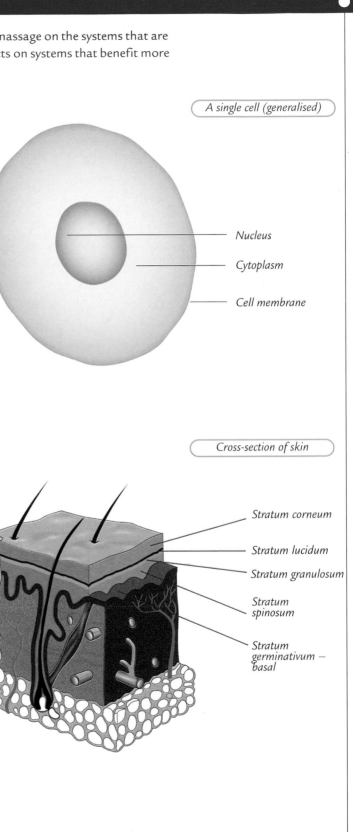

A single cell (generalised)

Nucleus

Cytoplasm

Cell membrane

Cross-section of skin

Stratum corneum

Stratum lucidum

Stratum granulosum

Stratum spinosum

Stratum germinativum – basal

EFFECTS AND BENEFITS OF MASSAGE

The muscular system

Massage has a direct effect on the muscles. The pumping action helps remove lactic acid, which builds up in overworked or over-exercised muscles, and toxins, thus reducing fatigue and stiffness. Massage improves circulation, which results in quicker delivery of nutrients and oxygen to muscles and faster removal of waste and carbon dioxide which helps muscles to function at their optimum level. Manipulation of muscle leads to relaxation and lengthening of that muscle, improving flexibility and range of movement. Massage also reduces muscle spasms and twitching by reducing the anxiety and tension which causes them.

Cross-section of a muscle

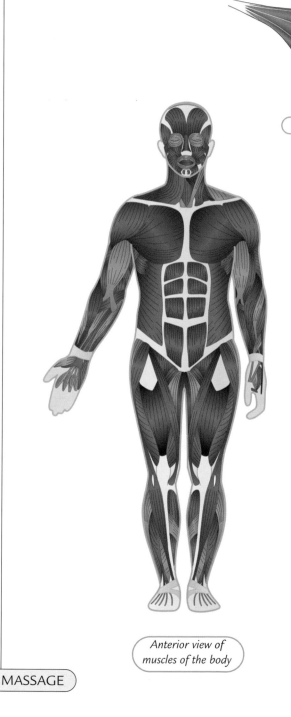

Anterior view of muscles of the body

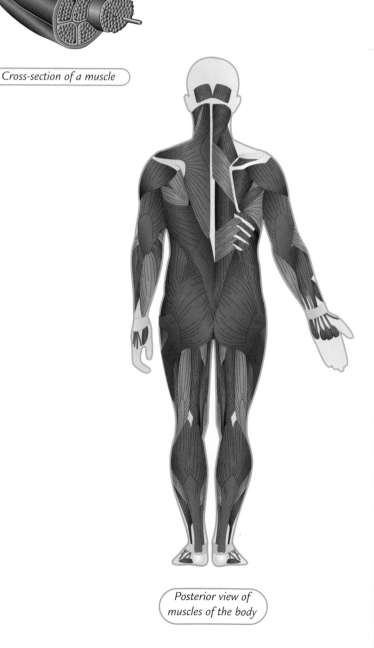

Posterior view of muscles of the body

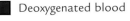

The circulatory system

Without a continuous blood supply, cells die and the body deteriorates rapidly. The pumping action of massage improves circulation, speeding up the movement of blood in the veins and arteries. Wherever possible the therapist assists the heart by applying pressure towards it. Oxygen and nutrients are delivered more quickly, waste removal is faster and the body therefore functions more efficiently. A gentle massage could lower high blood pressure by reducing the tension which can cause this condition.

■ Oxygenated blood

■ Deoxygenated blood

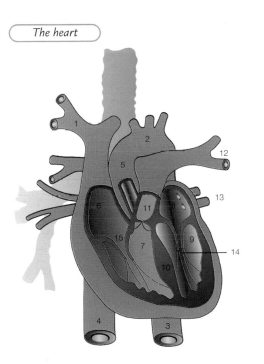

The heart

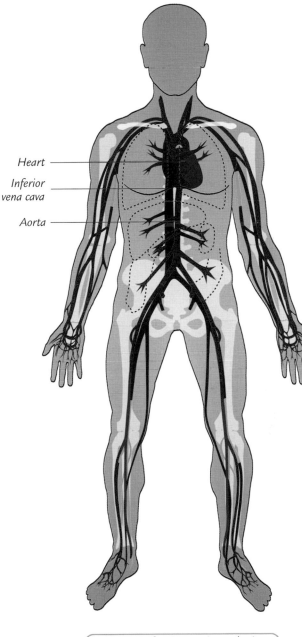

Heart

Inferior vena cava

Aorta

Overview of main arteries and veins

Key

1. Superior vena cava
2. Aortic arch
3. Descending aorta
4. Inferior vena cava
5. Aorta
6. Right atrium
7. Right ventricle
8. Left atrium
9. Left ventricle
10. Septum
11. Pulmonary valve
12. Pulmonary arteries
13. Pulmonary veins
14. Mitral (bicuspid) valve
15. Tricuspid valve

The lymphatic system

Unlike the blood, the lymphatic system has no pump to help it move lymph around the body. Massage is thus very helpful in supporting lymphatic functions, e.g. removal of waste and boosting immunity. It helps reduce swelling (oedema) caused by too much fluid in cells, reduces cellulite and improves lymph circulation. Lymphatic drainage massage, a type of massage used specifically to treat the lymphatic system, is discussed in Chapter 8.

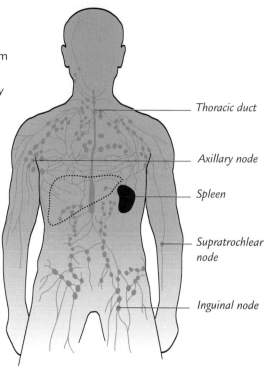

- Thoracic duct
- Axillary node
- Spleen
- Supratrochlear node
- Inguinal node

Overview of the lymphatic system showing lymph nodes and spleen

The structure of a nerve cell

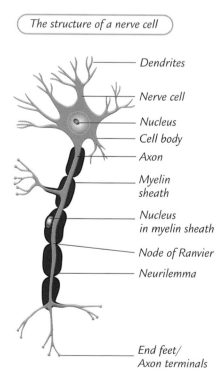

- Dendrites
- Nerve cell
- Nucleus
- Cell body
- Axon
- Myelin sheath
- Nucleus in myelin sheath
- Node of Ranvier
- Neurilemma
- End feet/ Axon terminals

The nervous system

Massage consists of several different techniques, some of which are invigorating whilst others are more relaxing. The effect of a massage on the nervous system will thus depend on the techniques used and the desired goal. For example, a massage to loosen up an athlete before an event is likely to be more stimulating than a massage used to relax a stressed executive. Thus massage can stimulate or relax the nervous system. A massage focused on stimulation will invigorate and wake up the nerves, energising the body. A more relaxing massage will calm the nerves, helping to release tension, stress and promote relaxation.

Other benefits

The following systems all benefit from massage but the effect is more indirect. For example the skeleton will feel less stress because the muscles have been massaged and are working more efficiently.

The skeletal system

The beneficial effects of massage on the muscular system have a positive knock-on effect for the skeleton. The soothing, stroking effleurage techniques of massage help to reduce stiffness and immobility around joints whereas improved muscle flexibility and tone reduces any strain on the joints and bones and improves posture.

The skeleton: anterior view

Side view

The digestive system

Massage encourages better digestion and assimilation at every level of body function, whether in a cell or in the stomach. It does so by improving the circulation, thus speeding up the delivery of nutrients. It also improves elimination by speeding up the removal of waste and increasing the flow of blood to the liver. Also by improving muscle function it helps strengthen the muscles of the abdomen thus assisting peristalsis and preventing constipation and/or flatulence.

Salivary glands

Tongue
Mouth
Oesophagus
Stomach
Liver
Large intestine
Small intestine

The digestive system

EFFECTS AND BENEFITS OF MASSAGE

The respiratory system

Massage is very relaxing and when relaxed the body can breathe more easily and deeply. This enables better absorption of oxygen and more efficient removal of carbon dioxide. In addition, the muscles involved in respiration (the diaphragm and intercostal muscles) will be less tense and thus function more efficiently.

The urinary system

Massage encourages better waste removal at every level of body function. It thus encourages urine production and excretion which helps rid the body of toxins and excess liquid.

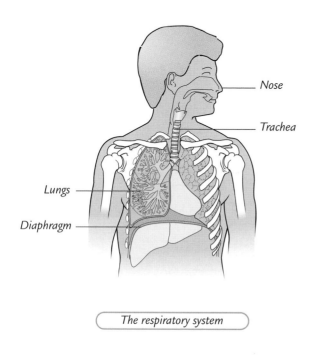

Nose

Trachea

Lungs

Diaphragm

The respiratory system

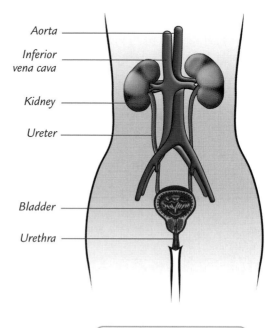

Aorta

Inferior vena cava

Kidney

Ureter

Bladder

Urethra

The urinary system (female)

GENERAL SUMMARY

Massage aids circulation, mobilises joints and muscles, improves digestion and by helping overall relaxation, improves and maintains general health.

You now know that massage benefits the whole body and its individual systems.

5 Professional conduct and consultation

In Brief

A massage treatment consists of using massage techniques to promote good health and relaxation. To do this a therapist must know how to find out as much as possible about the client's health and lifestyle so that treatment can be tailored to their requirements. This chapter explains consultation techniques and how to carry out a treatment. It also outlines how the therapist can take care of themself. Throughout this section the person receiving treatment will be referred to as the client.

Learning objectives

The target knowledge of this chapter is:
- professionalism
- hygiene procedures
- communication skills
- consultation techniques
- keeping client records
- contraindications
- where to give a massage
- required equipment
- how to ensure client modesty
- how to relax the client
- professional practice
- care of the massage therapist.

PROFESSIONALISM

Your appearance should confirm to your clients that you are a professional and qualified therapist and should give them the confidence to enable them to relax, knowing that they are safe in your hands. Within the first fifteen seconds of meeting, your client will make a number of judgements about you and your abilities, all of which will be based on your attitude and your appearance. For example, if you look untidy and dishevelled a new client may make the assumption that the service you will provide to them is going to be slapdash and careless. If, though, you look neat and well groomed, a new client is much more likely to assume that your treatments will be careful, competent and professional.

To ensure that you look professional throughout your working day you need to pay careful attention to the following:

1. Personal hygiene

Personal hygiene is a key element of professional presentation. Use a deodorant or anti-perspirant to prevent body odour. Check that your breath is fresh on a regular basis throughout the day. Also ensure that your hair is clean and tied back off the collar and face and that your nails are short, clean and without nail polish.

2. Uniform

A clean and freshly ironed uniform is essential to presenting a professional appearance. If you are working in a clinic you will be expected to wear professional work wear. If wearing white at work you will almost certainly need at least three uniforms; one to wear, one to wash and one to keep at work as a spare just in case you have an accident. Nothing looks more untidy or

unprofessional than a white uniform that is marked with splashes or stains. It's worth noting that, for reasons of hygiene, many employers will expect you to wear tights or stockings, even during the hot summer months. If you wear tights, do make sure that they are plain and a natural colour. If you are wearing trousers you should choose full, flat shoes and socks of the same colour. It is important always to make sure that you look neat and well groomed.

3. Hair

Hair must be clean and must be tied back from your face so that it doesn't flop forward onto your face, or rest on your collar. Tied back hair will be cooler and more comfortable for you, and will also be more hygienic for the client.

4. Nails and hands

Nails and hands must be kept scrupulously clean. Nails should be neatly trimmed, as this is essential to perform the massage techniques correctly. The client should feel the pressure of the treatment and not sharp nails pressing into their skin. Nails should also be unvarnished.

5. Perfume

Heavy perfume should be avoided as some clients may find strong odours unpleasant, or may even be allergic to certain fragrances.

6. Shoes

Shoes should be practical and, above all, comfortable as you will be wearing them throughout the working day. Your shoes should have closed toes and heels, and must be flat. As you are likely to be on your feet for long hours it's a good idea to ensure that you have a suitable pair that you can change into halfway through the day. This will help to keep your feet fresh and comfortable. It's also a good idea to have spare socks or tights to hand so that you can change those as well if you need to.

7. Jewellery

Jewellery must be kept to a plain wedding band and small stud earrings. Dangling earrings, bangles and rings must be avoided at all times as they are unhygienic and may even injure your clients. Wristwatches should be removed and left in a safe place until the end of the day, but fob watches may be worn on your uniform.

KEY POINT

Never, ever, chew gum or suck sweets whilst talking to, or working with, a client. This applies throughout the premises and, if you want to maintain the best impression with your clients, outside the premises as well

CHECKLIST

This checklist is a set of quick professional appearance checks that you can run through at the start of the day and before each client.

Before you meet your client
CHECK THAT:

- your personal hygiene is beyond question
- your uniform is spotless
- your hair is clean and neatly tied back from your face and collar
- your hands are freshly washed, and your nails are clean, neatly trimmed and filed and unvarnished
- you are not wearing heavy perfume
- your shoes are comfortable and clean, your socks are clean and your tights are not holed or laddered
- your jewellery is, at most, a plain wedding band and/or a pair of stud earrings.

A word about punctuality

Your client is entitled to expect that when they arrive for their appointment their therapist will be ready and available to begin the treatment. If you are late and keep your client waiting this sends a clear message that you do not consider them to be your number one priority. Many clients, quite rightly, will feel upset and irritated if their treatment doesn't start on time.

Also, your employer will expect you to complete a treatment within a commercially acceptable time. For example, in most clinics or spas, it is considered to be commercially acceptable to provide a massage treatment lasting for approximately one hour, and the price set for that treatment will be based on the cost of one hour of the therapist's time, plus the cost of clinic overheads such as lighting, heating, products used and so on. If, though, the therapist spends longer than an hour providing the treatment this will have an effect on the business – if fewer clients than expected are treated during the course of a day this means less money going into the till. This, in turn, will affect the employer's profits, and their ability to keep the business running successfully. In addition, clients often have busy schedules and plan carefully to fit a complementary therapy treatment into an hour. If the therapist draws out the treatment so that it takes longer than an hour, this can have a knock-on effect on the client's plans for the rest of the day, and make them late for other appointments. What should have been a soothing and relaxing experience can, if it takes too long, turn into a frustrating and irritating event, which spoils the remainder of the client's day. This is not good for the reputation of either the individual therapist, or the business. Keeping to time is an important part of professionalism. If you find that you are

Note:

- being professional is about earning and keeping the trust of your clients
- your appearance should confirm to your clients that you are a professional therapist whose personal hygiene and presentation is beyond question
- You should know the time allocated for each treatment, and stick to it
- if, for any reason, you have to keep a client waiting make sure that you apologise sincerely, and assure them that the delay was unavoidable and will not happen again
- if you find that you are running late on appointments, think about why it happens, and address the issue so that the delay is not repeated.

regularly running late with clients – which means keeping the next client waiting – you need to reflect on why this is happening, so that you can address the problem. These points also apply if you are self-employed or running your own complementary therapies center.

Some tips that can help you keep to time are to make sure that you do not:

- draw appointments out by chatting too much
- forget to keep an eye on the clock
- overestimate how much you can do in a given time.

Always remember that, after one client leaves, you will need a few minutes in which to prepare the treatment room – and yourself – for the next client.

THE PROFESSIONAL ENVIRONMENT

As well as making sure that your own appearance is immaculate, it's vital that you ensure that your treatment room, and everything in it, is spotlessly clean, neat, tidy and ready for the client's treatment. Needless to say, no client wants to find themselves in a treatment room, which looks untidy or unhygienic. And, from the client's point of view, nothing appears less professional than settling down for a treatment only to find that the therapist has to leave the room to gather extra supplies such as towels or treatment products.

CHECKLIST
As one client leaves and BEFORE the next client arrives CHECK THAT:

- the treatment room is spotlessly clean, neat and tidy
- you have opened windows to allow in fresh air (if possible), or used an air freshener, if necessary
- any bins are emptied before the next treatment
- your equipment trolley is clean
- you have sufficient supplies of all the products you need for the next treatment – e.g. fresh towels, tissues, cotton wool, treatment media, etc.
- any equipment you intend to use is clean (and sterilised where necessary) and in perfect working order
- you have your client's records to

hand or, for a new client, you have a new record card ready to be completed
- you have checked around the room to make sure that, in your professional opinion, everything is in order and ready for the next client.

The client will judge the quality of the service you provide on their complete experience with you. Even if the treatment you provide is perfectly satisfactory, if a client judges that some other aspect of the environment is unacceptable – for example, unhygienic or untidy – then they'll probably look around for another clinic that provides a cleaner, more pleasant, more comfortable setting for their next treatment. In other words, you are quite likely to lose a client to another business.

Hygiene
Providing a hygienic environment is a duty we have to our clients. It is also, for your clients, an important criteria by which they will judge your services, and whether, or not, to return or to recommend you to their friends and acquaintances. Good clinic hygiene is a continuous process that will, if carried out properly, ensure that all of the treatment areas, and all equipment used within it, are clean and free from

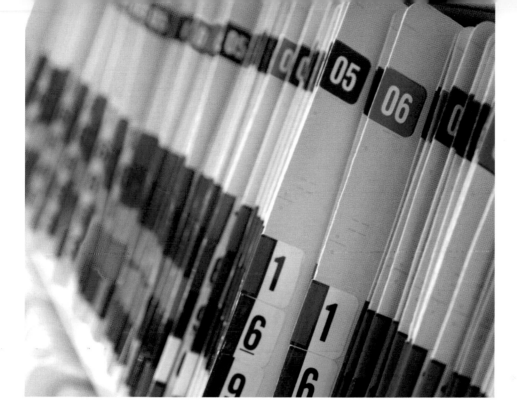

contamination. Preventing infection means ensuring that microorganisms (organisms that are so small they cannot be seen with the naked eye) such as bacteria, viruses and fungi do not have the opportunity to survive and multiply.

Bacteria

Bacteria are tiny and have a range of shapes – round, rod-like, or flagellate – and are only about one thousandth of a millimetre across, with millions living in a teaspoon of sour milk. While bacteria can play a beneficial role in parts of the ecosystem, may even provide antibiotics, and can help with our digestion, they are a cause of diseases ranging in severity from upset stomachs to pneumonia, tuberculosis and typhoid fever.

Viruses

Viruses are about a tenth the size of bacteria – indeed there is even one group, called bacteriophages, that feeds upon bacteria. They are responsible for some of the most devastating diseases of plants and animals. In humans, they are responsible for ailments from the common cold to herpes and HIV.

Fungi

While fungi can be seen (and enjoyed) as mushrooms, they are generally microscopic, and are another infectious organism that may affect our clients and us. They are responsible for the rising of our bread and the production of Penicillin, but they are also the causes of ringworm, thrush or candida, athletes' foot (tinea pedis) and fungal nail infections.

Parasites

Humans may play host to a number of parasites – organisms that use us for food, growth and shelter. They can live in the digestive tract as intestinal worms or on the body as lice - pediculosis capitis, corporis and pubis which are found in the skin and hair. Another parasite, the scabies or itch mite, burrows into the skin and feeds on blood. Parasites can cause ill health through cross infection – scratching infected areas.

Type of infection	Characteristics	How it spreads	Examples
Bacterial infection	Caused by bacteria, which are single-celled micro-organisms	Bacteria reproduce at the site of the infection – skin, ear, throat, vagina etc.	Skin infections such as impetigo (staphylococcus pyogens) or acne (propionibacterium acnes) Food poisoning such as salmonella
Viral infection	Caused by viruses, which are micro-organisms smaller than bacteria. Viral infections do not respond to treatment with antibiotics – penicillin etc.	Viruses reproduce inside human cells	Common cold Cold sore – herpes simplex Chicken pox – herpes zoster Wart – verrucae Hepatitis A and B HIV, which can lead to AIDS – Acquired Immune Deficiency Syndrome
Fungal infection	Caused by parasitic growth, which includes moulds, rusts, yeasts and mushrooms	Fungus is reproduced by spores	Ringworm – tinea pedis, capitis or corporus Thrush – candida albicans
Parasitic infestation	Caused by microorganisms that live on human tissue such as blood and keratin.	Spread by contact	Lice – Pediculosis capitis, corporis, pubis; Scabies (Sarcoptes scabiei)

The client can pick up an infection from equipment that has not been properly cleaned and sterilised, or from products that have deteriorated with age or have been contaminated by another client. To prevent the spread of bacteria, viruses, fungus or parasites within your working environment it's vital that you take the utmost care to ensure thorough sterilisation and sanitisation. This will ensure that no cross-infection occurs between one client and another. A variety of sterilisation methods and techniques are available for use in the salon. Here are some of the most suitable.

Autoclave

An autoclave is an item of electrical equipment which is used to sterilise small metal items of equipment such as, for example, scissors. When water is heated at normal atmospheric pressure, it boils at 100 degrees centigrade. The autoclave heats water under pressure, which increases the temperature at which the water boils. At a pressure of 15 pounds per square inch (psi) the boiling point of water is raised to over 120 degrees centigrade – a temperature at which good sterilisation can be achieved in 20 minutes. An autoclave, especially one with an automatic timer and a pressure

TEMPERATURE REGULATOR

gauge, is simple and effective to use and economical to run. Items to be sterilised must be capable of withstanding the heat in the autoclave, and this method is very suitable for metal instruments. It is vital that all items are washed or wiped prior to being placed in the autoclave to ensure that all surfaces are free to be cleansed.

Disinfectant liquids and solutions

We are all familiar with the use of disinfectant liquids and solutions in the home, and appropriate products have a valuable role to play in the hygiene and safety of our clinics. In clinic use, a disinfectant must be effective, economical to use and inoffensive. Typical professional products are either chemical disinfectants that may require dilution according to their instructions for use, or alcohol-based disinfectants that may be used in the form of liquids, wipes, or gel-based hand washes. Examples include products such as Barbicide, or Milton.

Before using any disinfectant product remember to:

- select an appropriate product for the use to which you are putting it
- clean small tools before disinfecting
- follow the instructions

- wear appropriate safety equipment
- allow enough time for the product to work.

After use, remember that used products will be contaminated and no longer effective, and so should be disposed of carefully. Also bear in mind that some products, such as alcohol/gel hand cleansers may be flammable.

Ultraviolet radiation (UV)

Short wave ultraviolet radiation can be used to sanitise small items. The article to be sanitised is placed in the UV cabinet but must have already been cleansed.

The UV radiation kills micro-organisms on the surface of the article. The UV radiation is only effective on the surface of items being sanitised (as it cannot pass through them) and, as light travels in straight lines, items must be turned during the process so that all surfaces are brought into the light and out of the shadow. The process takes roughly twenty minutes, and has the added benefit of not heating the item.

Chemical sterilisers

Liquid chemical sterilisers are plastic boxes or containers, usually with a perforated tray on their base. Most clinic materials can be sterilised by cleaning and drying them thoroughly and then immersing them in the liquid chemical in the steriliser. After the time indicated on the chemical manufacturer's instructions (usually between 10 and 30 minutes), the items can be removed and should be thoroughly rinsed. It is very important to choose the correct chemical for your sterilisation needs. The chemical liquid requires changing after the time specified by the manufacturer, usually about 14 to 28 days. Be very careful to avoid skin contact with the chemical liquid.

Hot bead steriliser

Hot bead sterilisers are small and easy to use. They are suitable for sterilising small objects but not for brushes, plastic, sponge or glass. Tiny glass beads are contained in a protective insulated case and heated to between 190 and 300°C (375-570°F) as indicated by the manufacturer. Sterilisation takes between 1 and 10 minutes

How infections spread

Infections are spread by touch, food and water droplets in the air, and through contact with cuts and grazes and other kinds of skin abrasions. Although it is almost impossible to create a completely sterile environment, you can reduce the risk of spreading infection by:

- not treating clients who have an obvious infection or, if the area infected is small, by avoiding it
- sterilising equipment
- disposing of waste safely
- maintaining the highest standards of hygiene

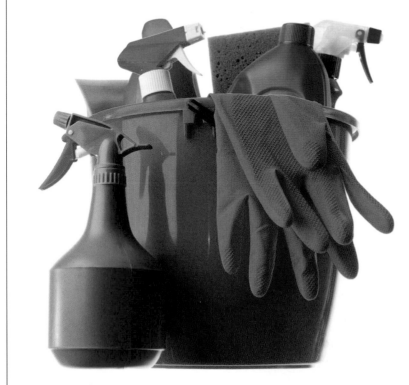

CHECKLIST
Ways to ensure a professional level of clinic hygiene

- All hard surfaces – floors, worktops, trolleys, toilets, washbasins etc – should be daily washed down with a disinfectant /sanitiser
- Clean bed linen should be used for each client, or the treatment couch or chair should be covered with clean couch roll for each new client
- Clean towels must be provided for each client, and towels should be laundered daily
- Clean towelling robes (if used) should be provided for each client
- Towels, blankets, towelling robes etc. should be laundered daily and then should be stored, clean, in a closed cupboard or laundry bin
- Waste bins should be emptied after each client and at the end of each day and disinfected
- Broken glass should be disposed of in a sharps container as the contents are collected and professionally incinerated.
- If a client has any open wounds or abrasions on their skin you should avoid touching these areas, and should make sure that the wounds are covered with a plaster before the treatment starts.
  The same applies to the therapist. Cross infection between clients can be prevented by:
- using disposable spatulas – for treatment media removal i.e. creams from pots etc
- never using fingers to decant products
- not scraping back into the main container any product that has been in contact with either your hands or any part of the client
- Used cotton wool, tissues etc. should be immediately disposed of in a covered waste bin

- Washing your hands thoroughly before and after every treatment is a must.

Thorough hand washing means:
- using an antibacterial soap or bactericidal gel and warm, running water
- washing forearms, wrists, palms, backs of hands, fingers, between fingers and under fingernails
- rubbing hands together for at least 10-15 seconds
- using a clean towel, or a disposable paper towel.

CHECKLIST
Health and hygiene terms you should know
- **Antiseptic:** a chemical used to reduce the growth of bacteria
- **Asepsis:** clean and free from bacteria
- **Disinfectant:** chemical used to destroy bacteria not their spores
- **Non-pathogenic Bacteria:** bacteria which is harmless or even beneficial to the human system – for example: Lactobacillus acidophilus which is found in yogurt, and Lactobacillus casei which is found in many cheeses
- **Pathogenic Bacteria:** bacteria which

is harmful and which causes diseases such as, for example, cholera, typhoid and tuberculosis
- **Sanitise:** make clean
- **Sepsis:** severe illness caused by overwhelming infection of the bloodstream by toxin-producing bacteria, which can originate anywhere in the body
- **Sterilise:** make clean and completely free from bacteria and their spores

KEY POINTS
- infections caused by bacteria, viruses, fungi and parasites can easily spread from one client to another
- a client can pick up an infection from equipment that has not been properly cleaned and sterilised, or from products that have been contaminated by an infected client
- good clinic hygiene is a continuous process
- thorough hand washing is essential to good hygiene as it will prevent the spread of any infection, and keep you and your clients safe.
- Using a hand cream after washing will soothe skin and prevent dryness

PROFESSIONAL COMMUNICATION

As a massage therapist good communication skills are at the heart of your ability to relate to your clients and to deal with them professionally. By using good communication skills you will encourage your client to relax in your care.

These skills include:
- asking the right kinds of questions
- listening with attention and interest
- being comfortable with silence
- using appropriate body language.

This, in turn, will contribute to their enjoyment of the treatment and should,

encourage them to return.
Asking questions is one of the best ways of encouraging clients to communicate with you and give you the information you need to treat them effectively.
When asking questions it's important to understand the difference between closed and open questions, so that you can ask the right kind of question at the appropriate time.
Closed questions are those to which your client will be able to give a short Yes or No answer.

Examples of closed questions include:
'Shall I open the window to let some air in?'
'Are you warm enough?'
'Would you like another blanket?'
'Have you had a facial massage before?'

Open questions can't be answered with a Yes or No. Open questions invite your client to provide information and to answer in detail.

Examples of open questions include:
'What do you hope the treatment will achieve for you?'
'Tell me about how you sleep?'
'Which parts of your back are most stiff and sore?'
'Tell me about your diet?'
'How have you been feeling since the last treatment?'

KEY POINT
Open questions are particularly useful when:
- you are meeting a client for the first time and need to take their history and complete their client record card
- you are talking to a client you have seen before and you want to find out how they responded to the last treatment you gave them and if there have been any changes, problems or improvements

Listening with attention and interest

Listening to your clients with genuine interest and attention will put your client at ease and will help to build a good professional relationship between the two of you. On the other hand, not listening to your client may persuade them that (1) you are not interested in them, (2) you don't care whether or not the treatment you provide is appropriate for their needs, and (3) you do not have a professional attitude to the work you do. Listening with attention and interest involves:
- being focused on your client throughout the time they are with you and concentrating on what they are saying
- listening without interrupting
- making eye contact with your client whilst they are speaking
- asking open questions to find out more
- remembering things your client has said to you so that at the next appointment you ask them about what they have told you – their planned holiday, family wedding, changes at work, new pet and so on

Being comfortable with silence

Some clients will enjoy talking throughout their treatment. They will regard the communication between you and them as an important part of the process, and they will happily chatter away about family and work and holidays and, probably, every other topic under the sun. Other clients, though, will regard their treatment time as a little oasis of peace and silence where they can simply relax and enjoy their therapy without having to make the effort to talk. Once you have obtained any information necessary from the client, for example: - 'How have you been?'; 'Are you warm enough?' 'Would you like more support under your knees?' - if the client lapses into silence, don't feel that you need to make small-talk conversation. This may be the only time during a busy working week when your client has the opportunity to completely relax and allow themselves to drift in peace and quiet.

However, during the massage treatment there will be times when you need to confirm tense areas that you are feeling, so you may need to ask further questions if they are conscious. You will also need to note non-verbal signs of discomfort, such as fidgeting and sighs.

You must be responsive to the needs of your clients.

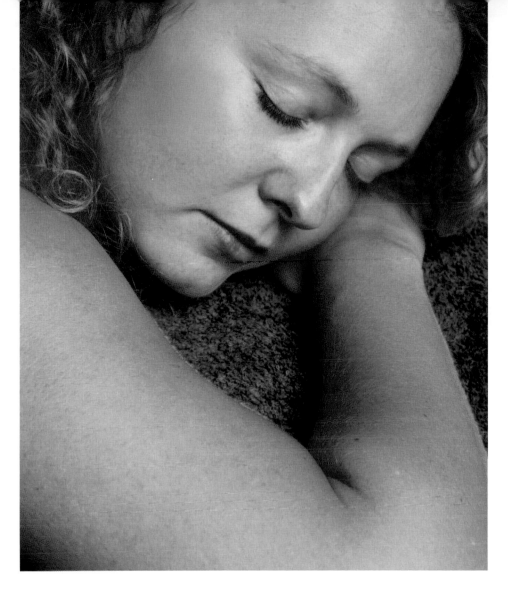

Using appropriate body language

It is really important that you use appropriate body language with your clients, as this will put them at ease and reassure them that they are in the hands of a professional therapist.

Non-verbal communication is another phrase for body language.

The elements of good communication are being able to:

- ask the right kinds of questions
- listen with attention and interest
- be comfortable with silence
- use appropriate body language
- make yourself clearly understood.
- open questions are used to gather information, whereas closed questions are used to elicit a simple 'Yes' or 'No' answer

Remember:

- listening with attention and interest will put your client at ease and make them feel valued and respected
- using positive and encouraging body language will help your client to relax and enjoy their treatment
- paying careful attention to your client's body language will help you to see when, even if they don't say anything, they are feeling uncomfortable or ill at ease with the consultation or treatment techniques i.e. pressure

CONSULTATION AND TREATMENT

HOW TO CARRY OUT A CONSULTATION

What is a consultation?

Before treatment can begin the therapist must find out why the client has come for massage and what their expectations are. This is a consultation and it serves as a fact-finding mission for both parties. The therapist must find out about the client's medical history, whether there are any contraindications to treatment and the client's reasons for choosing massage treatment (e.g. is it for a physical problem such as a muscle or joint problem, or poor circulation, for stress or anxiety or simply for relaxation purposes?). The client can find out what the treatment involves and whether it is suitable for their requirements.

As the first contact between therapist and client, the consultation also helps establish a professional relationship. This is especially important with massage treatment because the client must undress and may feel a little uncomfortable about this at the first session. The therapist can reassure the client about any aspect of treatment that concerns them, thus helping an anxious client to relax.

A consultation should cover the following information:

- the client's expectations, and whether these are realistic
- what the treatment involves and the possible effects (i.e. dispelling any unrealistic expectations)
- personal details: name, address, telephone number, date of birth, GP's name and address
- medical background: medicines being taken; medical conditions (any contraindications or problems should be referred; whatever the presenting problem a disclaimer form should be sent to the GP for confirmation that massage will not have any adverse effects); previous illnesses or hereditary diseases; operations; allergies.
- diet and other factors: eating habits, fluid and alcohol consumption, smoker or non-smoker, sleep problems (like insomnia)
- integral biology: work environment, family environment, lifestyle (sedentary or active).

Where do I record the information?

A therapist should keep records of each client's personal details, medical history and treatments. Record-keeping enables a therapist to keep track of a client's progress and the effect of treatment. It is also necessary to prevent abuse of the professional relationship, either by therapist or client. Each therapist will have their own system, e.g. index cards, pre-printed charts or a computer file. Examples of charts are shown opposite. Records should be kept in a locked place to ensure confidentiality. Records kept on a computer must comply with the Data Protection Act.

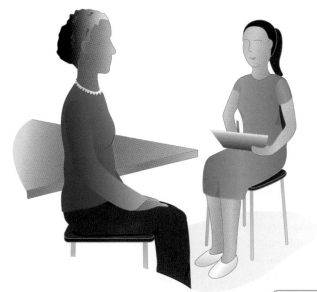

A consultation taking place

Client Consultation Form – Holistic

College Name:　　　　　　　Client Name:
College Number:　　　　　　Address:
Student Name:
Student Number:　　　　　　Profession:
Date:　　　　　　　　　　　Tel. No: Day
　　　　　　　　　　　　　　　　　　　Eve

PERSONAL DETAILS
Age group: ❑ Under 20　❑ 20-30　❑ 30-40　❑ 40-50　❑ 50-60　❑ 60+
Lifestyle: ❑ Active　❑ Sedentary
Last visit to the doctor:
GP Address:
No. of children (if applicable):
Date of last period (if applicable):

CONTRAINDICATIONS REQUIRING MEDICAL PERMISSION – in circumstances
where medical permission cannot be obtained clients must give their informed
consent in writing prior to treatment (select where/if appropriate):

❑ Pregnancy
❑ Cardiovascular conditions (thrombosis, phlebitis,
　hypertension, hypotension, heart conditions)
❑ Haemophilia
❑ Any condition already being treated by a GP or
　another complementary practitioner
❑ Medical oedema
❑ Osteoporosis
❑ Arthritis
❑ Nervous/Psychotic conditions
❑ Epilepsy
❑ Recent operations
❑ Any dysfunction of the nervous system (e.g. Multiple
　sclerosis, Parkinson's disease, Motor neurone
　disease)

❑ Bells Palsy
❑ Trapped/Pinched nerve (e.g. sciatica)
❑ Inflamed nerve
❑ Cancer
❑ Postural deformities
❑ Spastic conditions
❑ Kidney infections
❑ Whiplash
❑ Slipped disc
❑ Undiagnosed pain
❑ When taking prescribed medication
❑ Acute rheumatism
❑ Asthma
❑ Diabetes

CONTRAINDICTIONS THAT RESTRICT TREATMENT (select where/if appropriate):

❑ Fever
❑ Contagious or infectious diseases
❑ Under the influence of recreational drugs or alcohol
❑ Diarrhoea and vomiting
❑ Skin diseases
❑ Undiagnosed lumps and bumps
❑ Localised swelling
❑ Inflammation
❑ Varicose veins
❑ Pregnancy (abdomen)
❑ Cuts
❑ Bruises

❑ Abrasions
❑ Scar tissues (2 years for major operation and 6
　months for a small scar)
❑ Sunburn
❑ Hormonal implants
❑ Cervical spondylitis
❑ Gastric ulcers
❑ Abdomen (first few days of menstruation
　depending how the client feels)
❑ Haematoma
❑ Hernia
❑ Recent fractures (minimum 3 months)

WRITTEN PERMISSION REQUIRED BY:
❑ GP/Specialist　❑ Informed consent
Either of which should be attached to the consultation form.

PERSONAL INFORMATION (select if/where appropriate):

Muscular/Skeletal problems: ❑ Back ❑ Aches/Pain ❑ Stiff joints ❑ Headaches

Digestive problems: ❑ Constipation ❑ Bloating ❑ Liver/Gall bladder ❑ Stomach

Circulation: ❑ Heart ❑ Blood pressure ❑ Fluid retention ❑ Tired legs ❑ Varicose veins
❑ Cellulite ❑ Kidney problems ❑ Cold hands and feet ❑ Borderline low blood pressure 110/80

Gynaecological: ❑ Irregular periods ❑ P.M.T ❑ Menopause ❑ H.R.T ❑ Pill ❑ Coil
Nervous system: ❑ Migraine ❑ Tension ❑ Stress ❑ Depression
Immune system: ❑ Prone to infections ❑ Sore throats ❑ Colds ❑ Chest ❑ Sinuses
Regular antibiotic/medication taken? ❑ Yes ❑ No
If yes, which ones:
Herbal remedies taken? ❑ Yes ❑ No
If yes, which ones:
Ability to relax: ❑ Good ❑ Moderate ❑ Poor
Sleep patterns: ❑ Good ❑ Poor ❑ Average No. of hours
Do you see natural daylight in your workplace? ❑ Yes ❑ No
Do you work at a computer? ❑ Yes ❑ No If yes how many hours
Do you eat regular meals? ❑ Yes ❑ No
Do you eat in a hurry? ❑ Yes ❑ No
Do you take any food/vitamin supplements? ❑ Yes ❑ No
If yes, which ones:
How many portions of each of these items does your diet contain per day?
Fresh fruit:　Fresh vegetables:　Protein:　source?
Dairy produce:　Sweet things:　Added salt:　Added sugar:
How many units of these drinks do you consume per day?
Tea:　Coffee:　Fruit juice:　Water:　Soft drinks:　Others:
Do you suffer from food allergies? ❑ Yes ❑ No Bingeing? ❑ Yes ❑ No
Overeating? ❑ Yes ❑ No
Do you smoke? ❑ No ❑ Yes How many per day?
Do you drink alcohol? ❑ No ❑ Yes How many units per day?
Do you exercise? ❑ None ❑ Occasional ❑ Irregular ❑ Regular
Types:
What is your skin type? ❑ Dry ❑ Oil ❑ Combination ❑ Sensitive ❑ Dehydrated
Do you suffer/have you suffered from: ❑ Dermatitis ❑ Acne ❑ Eczema ❑ Psoriasis
❑ Allergies ❑ Hay Fever ❑ Asthma ❑ Skin cancer

Stress level: 1–10 (10 being the highest)
At work　At home

Example of client record

What are the contraindications to massage?

Massage is non-invasive, relaxing and natural. It is therefore generally considered a safe treatment for most people. However, there are two types of contraindications. Firstly, those that require written permission from a GP or medical specialist before massage can proceed. (In circumstances where permission from a third party cannot be obtained, the client must sign an informed consent stating that the treatment and its effect has been fully explained to them and that they are willing to proceed without permission from their GP or medical specialist.) And secondly, those that restrict massage treatment in the affected area or while the condition lasts.

Contraindications requiring written permission to proceed

- Pregnancy
- Cardio vascular conditions (thrombosis, phlebitis, hypertension, hypotension, heart conditions)
- Haemophilia
- Any condition already being treated by a GP or another complementary practitioner
- Medical oedema
- Osteoporosis
- Arthritis
- Nervous/Psychotic conditions
- Epilepsy
- Recent operations
- Diabetes
- Asthma
- Any dysfunction of the nervous system (e.g. Muscular sclerosis, Parkinson's disease, Motor neurone disease)
- Bell's Palsy
- Trapped/Pinched nerve (e.g. sciatica)
- Inflamed nerve
- Cancer
- Postural deformities
- Cervical spondylitis
- Spastic conditions
- Kidney infections

- Whiplash
- Slipped disc
- Undiagnosed pain
- When taking prescribed medication
- Acute rheumatism

Contraindications that restrict treatment

- Fever
- Contagious or infectious diseases
- Under the influence of recreational drugs or alcohol
- Diarrhoea and vomiting
- Skin diseases
- Undiagnosed lumps and bumps
- Localised swelling
- Inflammation
- Varicose veins
- Pregnancy (abdomen)
- Cuts
- Bruises
- Abrasions
- Scar tissues (2 years for major operation and 6 months for a small scar)
- Sunburn
- Hormonal implants
- Menstruation (abdomen – first few days)
- Haematoma
- Hernia
- Recent fractures (minimum 3 months)
- Gastric ulcers
- After a heavy meal
- Conditions affecting the neck

Does a contraindication mean that treatment cannot take place?

Not always. However, in the above cases and whenever you are unsure whether it is safe to proceed, it is best to refer the client to their GP for advice. The therapist should not, under any circumstances, attempt to diagnose a condition or decide whether an existing condition is treatable. The code of conduct of many complementary health associations states that diagnosis is not allowed. If there is any uncertainty, refer the client.

How and where do I carry out a consultation?

A consultation should take place in a comfortable, private room, where there is no chance of interruption. The room can be used for both consultation and treatment as long as it is possible to do so in a relaxed manner, i.e. do not sit behind a desk, and try to project an open, friendly image – keep arms and legs uncrossed, establish eye contact and smile. The client must feel reassured and comfortable in order to answer the questions and also to fully benefit from the treatment. Finally, the consultation should always take place when the client is fully dressed, not only because it prevents them feeling embarrassed or vulnerable, but also because it prevents the therapist feeling awkward if the treatment is contraindicated for the client and cannot take place. The consultation form should be re-checked at every appointment.

First impressions

Everything the therapist does communicates a message to the client and can affect the treatment. First impressions are very important, especially the first touch. If you choose to greet a client with a handshake remember that this is the first time you will touch them. A handshake that is limp, damp, sweaty, too firm or too weak may communicate to the client, either consciously or unconsciously, that the massage will have the same qualities. This could make them anxious or tense if they disliked the feeling. Be aware of this and act accordingly. Practice with friends to make sure that your handshake is relaxed and confident. If you have a tendency to sweaty palms use a light dusting of talc to counteract this. The first touch when beginning a massage is equally important: it needs to be firm, relaxed and smooth not ticklish, tentative or damp.

How do I get information from my client?

A new client may feel a little uneasy or nervous about the treatment, about being semi-undressed in front of a stranger or about revealing information about themselves. So your first task is to reassure and relax them by explaining what the treatment involves, how client modesty will be maintained through the use of towels and how all information will help you tailor treatment to their needs. You must also stress that all records are confidential. The next step is to encourage them to volunteer the required information. You will soon be able to judge how to approach this with different clients. For example, an open and relaxed person will need little coaxing but with shy, reticent clients a therapist will need to demonstrate listening skills. The following list of suggestions will help you get the most from a consultation.

- Start with general questions or, if you want to prompt , or sense a particularly shy client, use the form/record card as a starting point. Once you have begun asking questions which are easy to answer (name, address, date of birth etc) the more difficult ones about treatment and contraindications won't seem so daunting — the client will be in the rhythm of responding to your questions and will expect them rather than be made more nervous.
- Ask open not closed questions – ones that cannot be answered with yes or no. For example, ask 'What do you expect from a massage?' rather than 'Do you expect the massage to work?' or 'Tell me about your diet' rather than 'Do you eat healthily?'. No one likes to examine their own habits so it is best to address the questions in as open and unthreatening manner as possible.
- In order to instil trust, use your own body language to encourage and aid responses: nodding, smiling and leaning forward all communicate interest as does keeping eye contact. Looking away frequently, fidgeting or staring blankly will merely communicate nervousness and/or lack of interest, which will not help the client to feel confident in your abilities or your interest in them. Remember that, as a therapist, you are there to help the client. If you are unfriendly, nervous or uncommunicative the client is likely to pick up on this and react in a similar way.
- Be confident, enthusiastic and professional.
- Communicate your own belief and trust in the treatment – this will help the client to believe in it and will improve the psychological and physiological effects of the massage.
- Reassure the client that everything discussed will remain completely confidential and make sure that you never break this confidence.
- Treat everyone equally. If you cannot avoid bringing racist or sexist prejudices to the massage table then this is not the profession for you.

You now know how to carry out a consultation and find out the information needed to give an effective and safe massage. The next section explains how to carry out a treatment.

HOW TO CARRY OUT A TREATMENT

Where should a massage be given?

Massage requires the client to be partly or completely undressed (underpants should be kept on). The treatment room should therefore be private and without risk of interruption. Fear of someone entering the room will usually cause the client to tense up thus preventing or counteracting the positive, relaxing benefits of the massage. The room should have enough space for the couch and the therapist to move around it and work. It should also be the correct temperature, i.e. not too cold or too warm. You will be much warmer than the client because you will be exerting yourself physically. Make sure that there is a suitable ambient temperature. Towels should be neatly placed under and over the client, covering up any area of the body which is not currently being massaged. A blanket may be used on top of the towels at the beginning of the massage or during it, as necessary, to keep the client warm. The lighting in the room should be indirect and conducive to relaxation but bright enough to allow the therapist to work. Lamps with adjustable angles and brightness are preferable to glaring, overhead lighting.

What equipment is needed?

1) a massage couch

To perform a massage comfortably and effectively a height-adjustable couch covered with towels is recommended. Couch roll (disposable paper that can be pulled over the couch/towels) can be used to prevent the towels being stained by massage oil. If couch roll has not been used, the towels must be changed for each client. The couch should be firmly padded, to prevent the pressure of the massage being absorbed by soft cushioning under the body, easy to clean and wide and long enough to accommodate different clients. Some couches have a face hole, with a flap, to enable a client's head and spine to remain aligned when face down, but not all clients will require this or like it. Remember that the therapist should also be comfortable and not straining or overstretching to perform the treatment. A couch that can be adjusted to the right height for each individual prevents such problems. The couch should be at the therapist's hip height and the therapist should be able to extend an arm and comfortably place a hand, palm down, flat on the couch.

See also the 'Care of the therapist' section at the end of this chapter.

2) pillows and towels for support and protection

Pillows will help both client and therapist. For a massage on the back, pillows or rolled towels under the shoulders and ankles will help improve comfort. Using a face hole in the couch will help keep the head and spine properly aligned during a back massage. (However, not all clients will be comfortable using one.) Additionally, a pillow can be used under the chest for client comfort. For a front of the body massage a pillow under the neck and under the knees will provide support, relax the back and prevent strain. As mentioned earlier, towels are required to cover the parts of the client which are not being massaged.

3) couch roll (disposable paper)

Couch roll is optional. It can be used to protect towels from being stained by massage or essential oil.

4) changing facilities and bathroom

The client should be able to undress in privacy so adequate changing facilities will be required. Most local authorities also require that a shower should be available for client use. A large towel or robe should be provided for the client to wrap themselves in after undressing. Underpants should be kept on and spectacles/contact lenses and jewellery removed. It is advisable that both therapist and client go to the toilet before the massage begins to prevent interruption.

5) trolley

One or both hands should always be kept on the body during the treatment, since as soon as the hands are removed, the body registers this as the end of the massage and begins to 'change gear', waking up from the relaxation. Any form of interruption will disrupt the massage and lessen its positive effects. However, during the massage the therapist may need to reach the oil, cream or talc being used or extra towels. Ready-wipes or cotton wool and surgical spirit should also be available. A trolley stocked with the required equipment and moved around the room to convenient positions prevents unnecessary interruptions.

How do I ensure client modesty?

For most massage treatments, the client will need to undress to their underpants. A large towel or robe should be provided in the changing facilities for the client to wrap themselves in after undressing. Once on the couch, this large towel can be used to cover the upper body at the beginning and end of the massage. A second towel is used to cover the lower body. During treatment towels should be draped over the client, covering up any area of the body which is not currently being massaged. The towels help keep the client warm as well as ensuring that they do not feel exposed. At the end of the treatment the large towel can once again be used as a wrap for the body and the therapist should help the client off the couch so that they can hold on to the wrap.

How do I make sure the client can relax?

Hopefully, the client will feel more relaxed after the consultation. However, there are several other factors which can help. As discussed earlier, the room should be a comfortable temperature, the client's privacy should never be

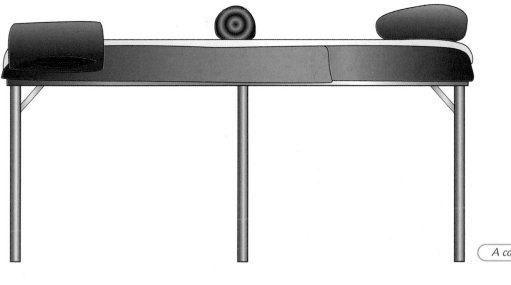

A couch set up for massage

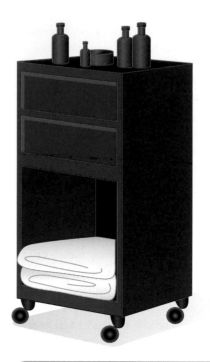

compromised and lighting should be
bright enough for the massage to be
carried out but soft. In addition, to make
the treatment as comfortable and secure
as possible there should be no chance of
interruption; windows should be
shielded with blinds or curtains;
changing facilities should open into the
treatment room or be positioned as close
as possible so that the client does not
have to walk very far once undressed. A
footstool or step may be placed by the
couch to enable the client to get onto the
couch without immodesty (this is
especially useful for elderly, shorter or
less flexible clients). Once installed on
the couch check that they are
comfortable and warm enough. Ask if
they wish to listen to music and if so play
something quiet and soothing rather
than loud and upbeat. Some clients may
prefer to talk, some may prefer silence.
Remember that this is their time and you
should respect their wishes — they are

Trolley set up for use during treatment

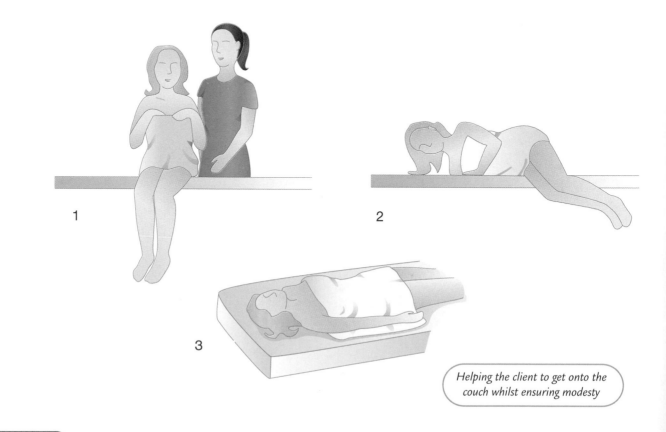

1

2

3

*Helping the client to get onto the
couch whilst ensuring modesty*

not paying to hear your views or personal preferences. During the massage listen to their comments, if any, and adjust the treatment accordingly, adding or reducing pressure or working on a particular area more if necessary.

What happens at the end of the massage?

Throughout the treatment you will have been using oil, cream or talc. At the end this needs to be removed from the skin. Most clients will simply choose to shower and wash off the medium. However, if for any reason this is not possible (because the client prefers not to shower rather than the shower not being available, which may contravene local authority regulations) or desirable, damp cotton wool should be used to remove the medium, followed by a skin toner and/or a hot towel.

Once this is completed, re-cover the whole body with the large towel and discreetly help the client to wrap themselves in it. When they are sitting up, help them off the couch. Once the client has dressed let them sit still for a moment, to give them time to 'wake up'. You may like to offer them a glass of water because massage often causes thirstiness, and water will help flush out released toxins.

Aftercare advice

After treatment many reactions can be experienced. You should explain to the client that this is a positive result of the treatment. Massage makes the body systems function more efficiently, speeding up waste removal and the elimination of toxins. Thus the after-effects may include:

- frequent urination
- headaches
- thirst
- sleepiness
- fatigue
- frequent bowel movements
- Nausea
- skin reactions
- healing crisis
- altered sleep patterns
- increased emotional state
- increased energy

Good professional practice

It is extremely important for any therapist to take the following information into consideration when performing a massage.

- **emotions and sex**

When carrying out a massage it is evident that the client will be semi-naked. His or her modesty is of paramount importance and a professional therapist will not allow any emotional or sexual involvement with the client to compromise the client's position. Vice-versa, if you feel that the client is behaving inappropriately towards you, you would be perfectly within your rights to discontinue the treatment.

- **psychology**

It is important not to become the client's counsellor. Obviously, if a client feels relaxed and comfortable with the therapist, he or she may discuss their personal matters but the therapist must resist the temptation to get involved, offering judgements or advice. It is also wise to avoid topics of conversation that may cause offence or strong feelings such as money, marriage, religion or politics.

- **hygiene**

The equipment (couch, trolley, towels, changing room and consultation room) should be kept clean at all times and the therapist should also pay attention to his or her personal hygiene since they will be spending intensive periods of time in a confined space with the client. Good hygiene is essential for ensuring a professional image and protecting the health of both therapist and client.

- **professional image**

The person giving the massage should be dressed comfortably in professional clothes and comfortable, flat shoes. Nails should be kept short, clean and unvarnished and jewellery avoided. Where

necessary, hair should be pinned or tied away from the face and off the collar.

You now know how to set up an area for giving a massage, how to ensure the client feels relaxed and comfortable and what constitutes good professional practice. The next section explains how the massage therapist can protect themselves whilst working.

THE USE OF MASSAGE IN A CARE SETTING

How can massage be used in health care?

Massage can benefit health on physical, psychological and pharmacological levels and is thus very suitable for use in a health care environment. When ill or hospitalised, one or more of the patient's five senses may be affected. Touch can enhance the life of a patient to great effect.

When is it not suitable?

Using massage in any way requires communication between the medical practitioner, therapist and patient. The therapist needs to know of any contraindications to treatment and prescription medicines the patient is taking. The massage therapist can ask the doctor to sign a letter of consent specifying the type of treatment to be performed. Some healthcare trusts decline written permission due to an increase in litigation but many doctors feel that their patients are able to take decisions about their own health.

What precautions need to be taken in this environment?

Therapists who are able to work in a care setting should be aware of and comply with any existing care plans, should keep detailed consultation and record forms and use massage with care and consideration.

Is massage suitable for people with special needs or learning difficulties?

The use of massage in this particular setting is becoming more widespread. Massage is often used in combination with specialised units such as Snoozelum rooms to enhance development and calm behaviour. Patients sometimes suffer physical problems caused by their repetitive or limited movements and massage has been used to help. Benefits include improved sleep patterns and a relaxation of physical tetany (muscle spasms).

Can massage be used with the elderly?

This sector of care is enlarging dramatically as more people live on into their 80s and 90s. The traditional role of the family as carers has changed and this task is now being undertaken by professionals. Massage is particularly applicable here as many elderly people often suffer the stress of bereavement, loss of their home, moving to a new area and making new friends coupled with ill health. Loss of physical contact also plays a large part as people age and become withdrawn as a result of change.

Can massage help the terminally ill?

Several programmes exist in hospitals and healthcare trusts where the importance of stress reduction, alternative pain relief and simple human contact have been recognised. Some general hospitals are also using massage for palliative care.

CARE OF THE MASSAGE THERAPIST

As you can probably tell from Chapter 3, massage is a very physical treatment. The effects of this treatment depend on the physical energy of the therapist performing it. If, for any reason, that energy is depleted by health problems or limited by incorrect posture then the treatment will be less effective. Furthermore, any therapist continuing to work without paying attention to posture and correct working positions will cause damage to their own body, both in the short and long-term. This section explains how massage therapists can take care of themselves, both in preparation for working and during treatment, in order to protect their health and carry out effective massages.

How can a massage therapist protect/take care of themselves?

In order to protect themselves, massage therapists should pay attention to the following four areas: posture, working position, attitude and exercise. Each one of these factors contributes to the positive effects of treatment and prevents the therapist from damaging themselves.

What is posture?

Posture is the way we position and hold our body.

How can it help the massage therapist?

Good posture is necessary both professionally and physically. When greeting and treating clients, a therapist must always be aware of how they are

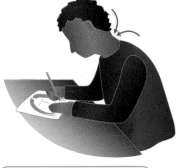

Incorrect sitting posture

holding themselves. This is both protective and demonstrative: many clients will have back and joint problems caused by incorrect posture and if the therapist is explaining how poor posture can cause these problems it helps if they themselves are following such advice. When consulting and working the therapist should avoid:

- tension in arms, neck and shoulders
- stiff, rigid legs and locked knees
- stiff, inflexible wrists and hands
- uneven distribution of weight in the legs, i.e. resting on one more than the other
- bending without using the knees
- bending the spine
- slouching or crossing the legs whilst consulting
- repeating the same movements: varying the routines helps prevent repetitive strain injuries
- overstretching across the couch.

All of the above can cause back and neck problems, muscle strain and repetitive strain injuries. Not only are they damaging, they also affect the therapist's attitude (see below), give a poor impression and prevent the most effective treatment.

What is the correct posture for massage treatment?

There is no absolutely correct posture because everyone's body is different. However, a therapist should:

- keep the back straight but not rigid
- keep wrists and forearms as straight as possible without locking them
- keep legs slightly bent
- use a wide stance
- keep shoulders relaxed; it is a common tendency to tense shoulders, holding them close to the ears.

Practice rolling them away from the ears and towards the ground in order to release this.

- move around the couch instead of overreaching and risking muscle damage.
- distribute the weight of the body evenly between both legs. Many of us tend to rest on one leg, overworking it and weakening the other.
- take regular breaks (though not, of course, during a treatment).
- use a height-adjustable couch positioned so that it is possible to extend the arms and place the palms of the hands flat on the surface of the couch without strain.
- be aware of their own body, where tension is held and what causes strain. Awareness of one's own body's limits will help prevent overstretching it.
- remember that it is often the tiniest movements which cause the most damage.

Why is correct posture important to the treatment?

Massage is a very physical treatment and correct posture helps the therapist perform to the best of their abilities without damaging themselves. If the therapist is evenly balanced, with weight evenly distributed through the legs and pelvis, flexible and relaxed, the massage will be smooth, rhythmic and relaxed. If the therapist is moving in a jerky or unbalanced way, often as a result of tension in the body or an uneven distribution of weight in the legs, the treatment will also be jerky. Furthermore, good posture enables the therapist to concentrate on the massage without worrying about their own body and whether they will be able to perform the movements.

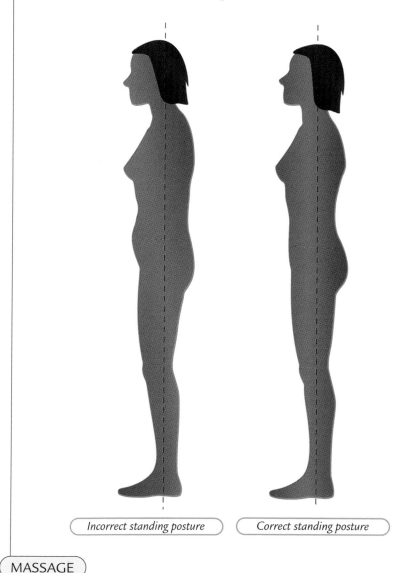

Incorrect standing posture   Correct standing posture

You now know why good posture is important to a massage therapist.

WORKING POSITION

What is a working position?

A working position is a stance adopted by the therapist whilst carrying out a treatment.

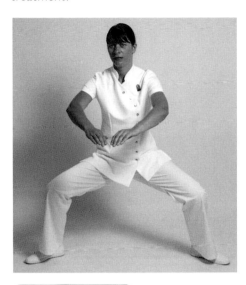

Side standing position

How does it help the therapist?

Working positions are designed to protect the working therapist from muscle or joint strain as well as allow maximum mobility and pressure for the treatment. The following working positions are recommended for full body massage.

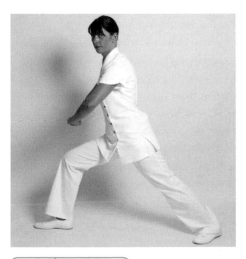

Striding position

- **Side standing position**

Place feet approximately 100cm apart with toes just under and in line with the edge of the couch and pointing out at 45 degrees, knees soft, hips forward, bottom tucked under, forearms at right angles to the body with wrists kept in alignment with arms and flexible. Be careful not to stiffen shoulders, knees or lower back and not to hang the head in order to look down. Keep the neck straight and look down from this position or, if this is not possible, tilt the head slightly by lowering the jaw rather than bending the neck. You can also have a wider stance and bend the knees more, to get closer to your client. This position is used for short strokes, such as petrissage and percussion, rather than effleurage, when work is across the muscles or on a local area not a whole section.

- **Striding position**

Stand with the body at an angle to the table, feet positioned as if striding forward, one in front of the other in a very wide stance/deep lunge. The knees need to be flexible not rigid and it is important to bend from the waist and not from the middle of the back. This position is used for strokes along the length of the body particularly the back and limbs. The therapist uses the striding position to push themselves forwards along the body. The weight is moved from the back foot to the front foot and this gives momentum to the stroke, as if the movement that the therapist should be making, given the position of the feet, is transmitted to the arms.

You now know how to position yourself when working.

ATTITUDE

What is attitude?

Attitude is the mental equivalent of posture. It is the disposition of the mind, how someone is thinking and feeling. Someone with a positive attitude is thinking and feeling positive.

Why is it important for the massage therapist?

Have you ever noticed that when you're in a good mood and you meet someone in a bad or negative mood, you often leave them feeling much less positive? This is because we are affected by other people's emotional moods and attitudes. When carrying out a massage a therapist's mood and attitude will affect their client. So a tense therapist will make the client tense, a hurried therapist will make the client feel rushed. A tense or hurried therapist is also more likely to damage themselves whilst working. If the massage is to have the desired effect, whether relaxing or energising, the therapist will need the right attitude. In general, the therapist should feel centred and focused, secure and calm and able to concentrate on using their own physical or mental energy to work on and improve the physical and mental energy of the client. Yoga, meditation and t'ai chi are all exercises for the mind and body which are useful for concentration and focus.

Exercise and breathing

A massage therapist will need to take regular exercise in order to have the physical fitness and stamina to carry out treatment. Exercise is also one of the best ways to relax after work, in order to prevent the build-up of tension and stiffness from working in similar standing positions all day. Hands and wrists should also be exercised on a regular

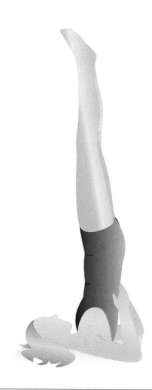

Yoga posture – a shoulder stand

basis to keep them supple and flexible. Finally, breathing exercises can help with relaxation both during and between treatments. Throughout the massage the therapist should be aware of their breathing and that of the client. They should encourage the client to breathe deeply and evenly and should make sure their own breathing is calm, regular and matches the client's pace. This will enable both parties to relax and concentrate on the treatment. Relaxation and breathing techniques are part of yoga, meditation and t'ai chi. It can be very beneficial for a massage therapist to themselves receive regular massage therapy.

You now know how to consult with a client and how to look after yourself as the therapist.

6 Using on-site massage to treat stress

In Brief

Massage is an holistic therapy because it treats the whole person. It is useful for treating stress and stress-related conditions because it helps to relax the body and reduce the effects of stress.

Learning objectives ●

The target knowledge of this chapter is:
● definition of the holistic approach
● definition of integral biology
● definition of stress
● how to use massage to treat stress.

THE HOLISTIC APPROACH & INTEGRAL BIOLOGY

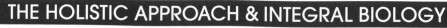

What is the holistic approach?

The term holistic comes from the Greek word 'holos' meaning whole. The holistic approach to treatment takes into account a person's whole being, not just the physical symptoms or problems but also psychology, environment and nutrition and the effects, both positive and negative, that these can have on the body as a whole.

What is integral biology?

Integral biology is the study of our environment's effect on our physical and mental health. Everything we do in our daily lives affects our bodies. For example, an uncomfortable working environment can cause stress, tiredness and related conditions, such as anxiety, depression and heart conditions. At home lack of exercise and a poor diet plus too much sedentary activity (watching TV, writing, reading, using computers) may cause similar problems.

What affects integral biology?

There are many factors that influence our integral biology. Some are negative and some positive.

Negative factors

- lack of exercise
- processed food
- chemically-treated fruit and vegetables
- lack of fresh air
- too much alcohol
- a stressful job
- bereavement or grief
- too much caffeine (tea, coffee, cola)
- lack of sleep
- financial problems
- worries about family/relationships
- too much time spent on or near electro-magnetic equipment (computers, photocopiers)
- a smoky or poorly ventilated home or office
- internalising problems and worries.

Positive factors

- regular exercise
- eating fresh (preferably organic or non-chemically treated) fruit and vegetables
- a varied and healthy diet
- drinking lots of water
- taking regular breaks at work and home
- reorganising work patterns to avoid sitting or standing in the same place for several hours in a row
- getting enough sleep
- getting plenty of fresh air and making sure a window is open when someone is smoking.

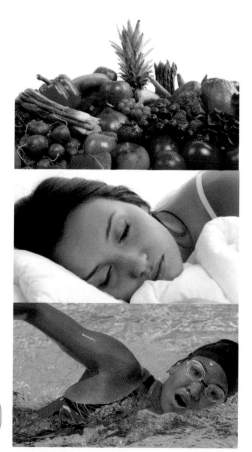

Good health depends on several factors including diet and rest.

Why is holistic approach important?

Because it treats each person individually and in the context of their own life. This enables people to improve their health themselves, thus re-establishing the body's equilibrium, known as

homeostasis. For the best therapeutic effect, all aspects of integral biology need to be considered.

You now know about the holistic approach and integral biology. The next section explains stress and how massage can be used to combat it.

STRESS

WHAT IS STRESS?

Stress is any factor that threatens our physical or mental well-being. Such factors can be imagined (worry about the future) or real (financial problems). It is not the factor itself that is damaging but the response to it. Some people have very stressful lives but manage stress so that it does not affect them whereas for others even the slightest worry can have damaging consequences.

There are two types of stress, positive and negative. Positive stress is necessary for some people because it helps them perform to the best of their abilities. For example, most actors and sportspeople will feel, and need, stress before a big performance or event and rather than hinder them, this positive stress helps them to concentrate and focus on the important moment ahead. Negative stress, however, is any factor which causes us to respond by worrying, panicking or losing our concentration.

How does stress affect us?

The body has always had to respond to stress. Thousands of years ago, stress factors were more physical. Humans needed to hunt for their food, protect themselves from wild animals and secure shelter. In the twenty-first century stress factors are likely to be more intangible, e.g. job insecurity, worrying about relationship difficulties or irritation about traffic jams. However, the effects of stress are exactly the same whether the

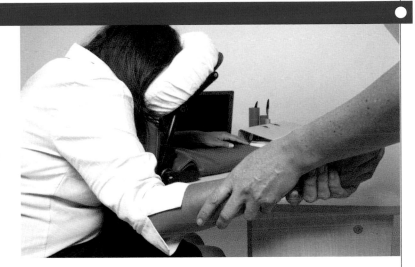

threat is an angry boss or an angry buffalo! The body, perceiving danger, prepares to face it or run away (the fight or flight syndrome). Several systems shut down and the body works to conserve energy to enable movement and escape. Adrenaline rushes into the body to warn of impending danger and the heart rate increases, the blood vessels contract increasing blood pressure, the digestive functions shut down and the muscles contract.

If the perceived danger is then either removed or escaped from, the stress response has achieved its aim and the body relaxes. However, usually, it is not easy to get away from the cause of the stress. Most stress factors are no longer responded to with activity. It is very hard for an office worker to run away from an annoying problem or colleague. As a result the body remains tense and cannot relax. It is this unused response mechanism which is damaging.

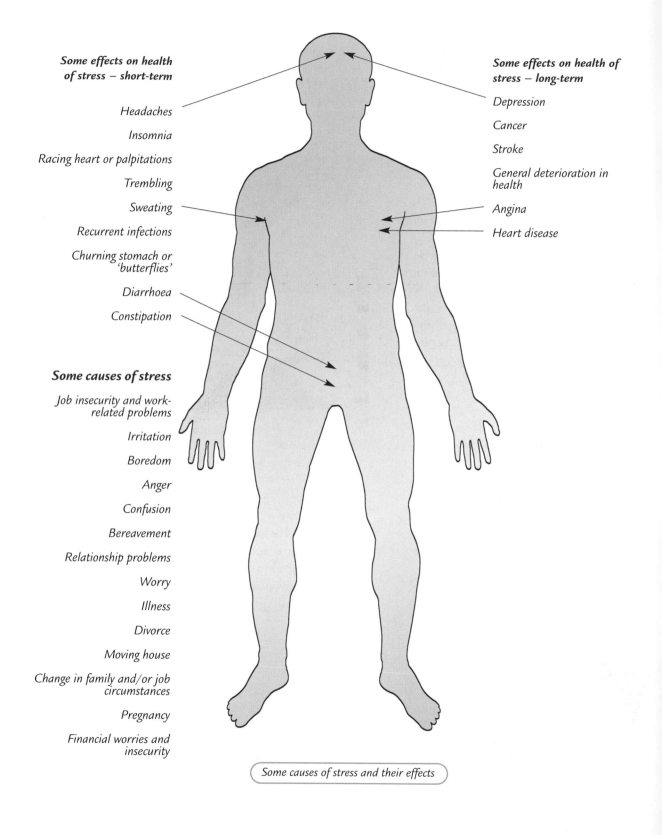

Some effects on health of stress – short-term

Headaches

Insomnia

Racing heart or palpitations

Trembling

Sweating

Recurrent infections

Churning stomach or 'butterflies'

Diarrhoea

Constipation

Some causes of stress

Job insecurity and work-related problems

Irritation

Boredom

Anger

Confusion

Bereavement

Relationship problems

Worry

Illness

Divorce

Moving house

Change in family and/or job circumstances

Pregnancy

Financial worries and insecurity

Some effects on health of stress – long-term

Depression

Cancer

Stroke

General deterioration in health

Angina

Heart disease

Some causes of stress and their effects

How is stress damaging?

It has been estimated that stress is the cause of 75% of disease. In the short term, as a response to perceived danger, stress is literally life-saving. If we didn't feel stress we would not make the effort to cross the road a little faster to get out of the way of an approaching car, or to perform to the best of our abilities to win a sports match or competition. However, in the long term, if a person continues to feel stress in response to external factors but does nothing either to remove the cause of the stress or to respond to it differently, the stress reaction can be damaging. The body remains in a state of alert and eventually this will have a physical effect on the systems concerned.

What are the symptoms of stress?

Anyone who has ever been nervous about an interview, exam, meeting or important sports event has felt some of the symptoms of stress. These include: churning stomach or 'butterflies', racing heart or palpitations, diarrhoea, loss of appetite, trembling, insomnia, sweating. In the medium term these symptoms, left untreated, may cause chest pains, allergies, persistent insomnia, high blood pressure, abdominal pain, migraines, depression, ulcers, asthma and infections. In the long term constant stress is known to cause heart disease, strokes, cancer and angina.

How can stress be cured?

Stress in itself cannot be 'cured' because threats to our well-being will always exist around us. However, it is not the threat but the way it is perceived and responded to that is most important. If stress is managed, it is no longer damaging, e.g. if stuck in traffic, one driver may become enraged whereas another will accept that this is a normal situation in a busy area. The first driver is responding to stress,

the second is managing it. However, the actual stress factor itself is the same.

How can stress be managed?

By learning to respond in a healthier way and using relaxation techniques. We cannot simply tell our bodies to relax; we have to learn how to relax them, via relaxing activities, such as walking, seeing friends or going to the cinema, as well as specific breathing, visualisation, relaxation techniques and massage.

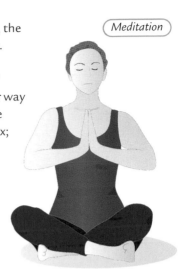

Meditation

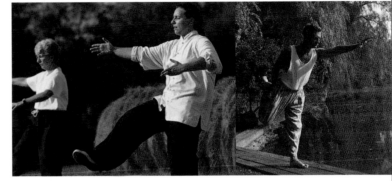

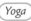

T'ai chi

Yoga

How can massage help?

When the body is stressed it must work harder than usual in order to remain balanced. Hence, stressed people tend to over-use conventional relaxation methods such as drinking and smoking in order to be calm. However, too much alcohol or nicotine can have an adverse effect on the body in the long run whereas an holistic treatment such as massage can help induce deep relaxation, helping to remove the pent-up tension of the stress response, without damaging the body. Furthermore, it is easy to forget what deep relaxation feels like and many clients are unaware of how much tension they hold in their body. By relaxing them properly, massage enables them to be more aware of what tension feels like

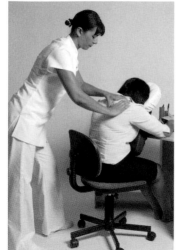

Using massage in the workplace

which in turn helps them to release it. Massage also enables the client to avoid stress altogether. When the body is relaxed problems and events tend to seem less daunting so the client will not feel as threatened and stressed, which in turn will prevent tension building up.

How does massage treat stress and its effects?

Massage treats stress in several ways:

- it is a treatment that relies on touch, one of the most neglected senses. The touch sustained through massage can boost self-esteem and comfort the lonely or bereaved.
- it boosts the immune system, which is weakened by constant stress, stimulates the circulation and the lymphatic system, increases energy levels and induces calm in both mind and body.
- it releases endorphins, the pain-relieving happy hormones.
- it stimulates the parasympathetic nervous system, which slows the body down, encourages deeper breathing, lowers heart rate and switches digestion back on.

- it relaxes all the systems of the body, which either shut down or speed up when stressed, and thus helps with stress-related conditions such as insomnia, headaches, backache and constipation.
- it helps treat depression and symptoms such as low self-esteem by boosting well-being which in turn increases self-worth.
- it stimulates the body's natural ability to repair and renew, at cellular level.

Massage for restoring health

Massage can be very useful as part of rehabilitation treatment after illness. Indeed, it has been used for this purpose for thousands of years, ever since the ancient Chinese used amma or massage for maintaining health. It helps to restore fitness and a sense of well-being. Illness weakens the mind and body but it often causes anxiety and insecurity as well, which themselves lead to stress and stress-related illnesses. Furthermore, long periods spent convalescing in bed can cause poor circulation, constipation, loss of muscle tone, stiff and sore joints and dull, congested skin. On a physiological level massage invigorates the body systems, which may have become sluggish or congested, stimulating poor circulation, boosting immunity, helping the removal of waste from the body, improving skin tone and elasticity and helping muscles recover their flexibility and strength. Psycho-logically, massage can help the client to feel less anxious about their health and regain a sense of well-being. All treatments should be approved by a GP, particularly after surgery.

You now know about the holistic approach and integral biology, stress and how massage can be used to combat it and help restore health after illness.

ON SITE MASSAGE SEQUENCE

Good posture and body position should be adopted according to the movement being given. The back should be straight at all times using good knee flexibility throughout. Repeats can be varied according to the time allowed.

The Back

- Standing behind the client tune in with the hands resting on the client's shoulders
- Circular effleurage down both sides of the spine together, working down from the shoulders to the hips and back up to the shoulders. Repeat twice.
- Petrissage with the heal of the hand pushing away from the spine working down from the top of the thoracic spine to the sacrum, sweep up lightly. The other hand rests lightly on the upper back. Repeat 3 times and then repeat on the other side of the spine.
- Effleurage back to the resting hand and place one hand on top of the other hand to do a sideways figure 8 effleurage from the shoulders to the hips and back again
- Slide one arm to the elbow position next to the top of the thoracic spine. With the elbow at 90 degrees straighten to 30 degrees and then return to 90 degrees, continue this petrissage movement working down the pressure points either side of the spine, first on one side of and then the other. Repeat twice both sides of the spine. Effleurage back to the shoulders
- Brisk rubbing either side of the spine with the sides of the hands. Work down the back and then up
- Effleurage with both hands down to one hip
- Knead around the hip and continue kneading up the side of the back to the

shoulders and return to the hips. Repeat other side

- Effleurage to the top of the trapezius
- Knead the upper back and shoulders
- Effleurage the upper back, shoulders, and around the scapula finishing at the lower border of the scapula
- Pressure points following the medial border of the scapula one at the lower end, one in the middle and one at the top. Work both sides together using the thumbs
- With forearms press down on the pressure points along the top of the trapezius. The first point is next to the neck, the next in the middle of the shoulder and last on the acromion process. Repeat 3 times. Begin lightly and gain pressure with each repeat.
- Effleurage down one arm to the wrist
- Hold the wrist bringing the arm to the side of the body, shake the arm and then bring the arm around the back of the body abducting the scapula.
- While supporting the arm with one hand the other hand uses deep effleurage around the abducted scapula followed by frictions around the medial border and posterior surface of the scapula.
- Effleurage the whole area to finish and then effleurage down the arm to the wrist.
- Holding the wrist, straighten then shake the arm and place it in its original position. Effleurage form the wrist up the arm and across the shoulders down the other arm to the wrist to repeat all massage movements on this side.
- Return to the back and begin double handed cupping be loosely clasping both palms together and using a back handed cupping movement over the shoulders and upper back. Continue with hacking

- Effleurage both sides of the back together starting at the shoulders covering the whole back effleurage down the neck and then up again.
- Effleurage to the shoulders and then squeeze along the top of the trapezius into the arms. Repeat 3 times

The Neck

- Single handed kneading on the cervical spine while supporting the top of the head. Continue to support the head throughout the back massage.
- Petrissage one side of the neck with the index and middle finger massaging up the cervical spine.
- On the same side work the pressure points along the base of the skull using the index and middle fingers and working from the base of the mastoid process to the occiput. Repeat once more.
- Repeat petrissage and pressure points on the other side of the neck and base of skull.

The Head

- Stroking from the top of the head to the neck covering the whole area
- Shampoo petrissage with both hands using all fingers and thumbs covering the scalp.
- Brisk rubbing with palms over one side of the head supporting the other side of the head. Repeat other sides
- Hacking two hands together over the head
- Stroking from the top of the head to the neck to finish.

The Arms

- Effleurage down one arm to the wrist, straightening and then shaking the arm
- Holding the wrist effleurage up to the shoulders and down to the wrist. Repeat 3 times
- Effleurage to the deltoids squeeze

down the arm to the wrist with both hands and then effleurage back to the deltoids. Repeat 3 times.
- Knead the upper arm followed by hacking the whole area
- Circular effleurage of the upper arm
- With the palm of the hand effleurage around the elbow
- Squeeze from the elbow to the wrist, effleurage back to repeat 3 times.
- On both sides of the wrist do a quick push-pull backwards and forwards with both hands.

The Hands

- With fingers squeeze the carpals and then the metacarpals 3 times.
- Thumb petrissage between each digit starting between the thumb and index finger massaging from the knuckles to the wrist. Repeat twice
- Using the thumb and index finger pinch and pull down between the metacarpals
- Petrissage up the thumb then pull and twist down and off followed by each finger in turn
- Hold the pressure point in the centre of the palm with one finger. Hold for 5 seconds
- Effleurage the arm and then stretch the arm holding the wrist
- Replace arm and effleurage from the wrist up the arm and across the shoulder down the other arm to the wrist to repeat all massage movements again.

To Finish

- Circular effleurage the whole back both sides together, starting at the shoulders, working down and then up the spine
- Sweep from the top of the head as far down the arms as possible and off the body
- Sweep from the top of the head down the sides of the back and off

- Sweep from the top of the head down the centre of the back and off
- Light feathering down the spine
- Hold the shoulders gently to indicate you have finished you massage.

50% OFF!
FULL ACCESS

DON'T FORGET NOW YOU CAN USE A RANGE OF ONLINE LEARNING RESOURCES FOR JUST £10 (NORMAL RRP £20)

The Massage e-Learning Resource has been designed to enhance your learning experience

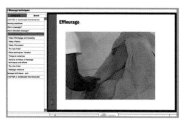

☐ Bring knowledge to life with videos of each technique as well as a full massage routine

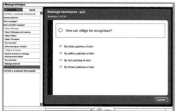

☐ Manage your learning with step-by-step modules and integrated 'classroom' sessions

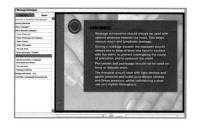

☐ Absorb information on key topics with interactive exercises and learning activities

To login to use these **e-learning resources**, visit **www.emspublishing.co.uk/massage** and follow the onscreen instructions

AN INTRODUCTORY GUIDE TO
Massage

7 What is Lymphatic drainage massage

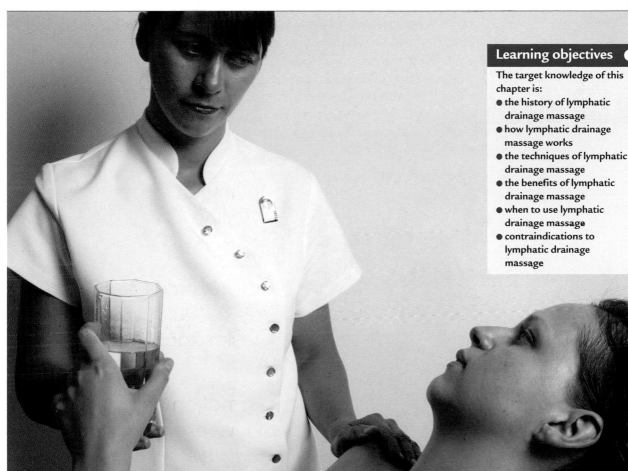

Learning objectives ⬤

The target knowledge of this chapter is:
- the history of lymphatic drainage massage
- how lymphatic drainage massage works
- the techniques of lymphatic drainage massage
- the benefits of lymphatic drainage massage
- when to use lymphatic drainage massage
- contraindications to lymphatic drainage massage

In Brief

Lymphatic drainage massage is a technique developed in the 1930s. It stimulates the functions of the body's secondary circulation, the lymphatic system, encouraging the removal and filtering of waste, toxins and excess fluids from cells as well as boosting the body's natural immunity.

WHAT IS LYMPHATIC DRAINAGE MASSAGE?

History

Lymphatic drainage massage was developed by Dr Emil Vodder and his wife Estrid in the 1930s. They worked as masseurs in Cannes in France and many of their clients were English people who had chronic colds and had come to the South of France to escape the damp in England which was considered to be aggravating their condition. Dr Vodder noticed that many of them had swollen lymph glands in their neck and although treatment of the lymphatic system was not recommended at the time due to the lack of knowledge about it, Dr Vodder decided to develop a system for treating it. They later established an institute in Austria.

What is lymphatic drainage massage?

Lymphatic drainage massage is a system of massage techniques that help the lymphatic system to function effectively.

What does it do?

Lymphatic drainage massage helps to boost the functions of the lymphatic system. It thus improves the circulation of

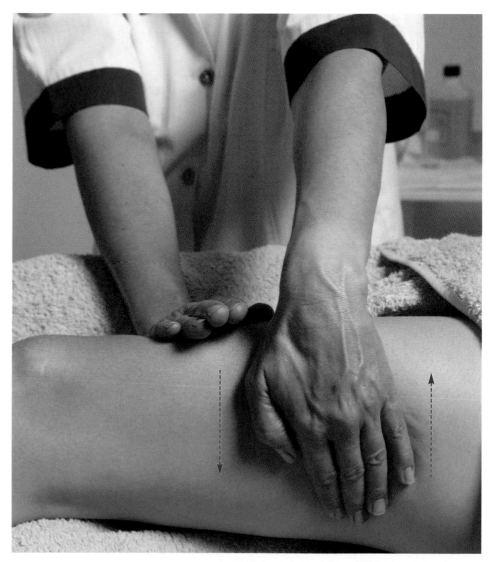

lymph which helps fluid drainage from cells and the elimination of waste, improves the production and distribution of antibodies and lymphocytes (a type of white blood cell) thus boosting immunity from disease and stimulates the lymphatic system's filtering process thus helping remove toxins and bacteria from the body. It also works on the autonomic nervous system, helping to slow the sympathetic nerves (which enable activity) and stimulate the parasympathetic nerves (which enable relaxation), thus helping relaxation and the reduction of stress.

When should it be used?

To clear congestion, waste and fluid from the system. It is thus indicated for:

- acne
- allergies
- cellulite
- fluid retention
- headaches/migraines
- menopause
- PMS
- respiratory congestion (catarrh)
- stress
- swelling (oedema)
- tiredness

When shouldn't I use lymphatic drainage massage?

Lymphatic drainage massage is contraindicated for:

- arthritis
- asthma
- Bell's Palsy
- cancer
- diabetes
- epilepsy
- heart and circulatory problems
- kidney problems
- lymphoedema
- menstruation
- nerve (inflamed)
- nerve (trapped)
- nervous/psychotic conditions
- osteoporosis
- pregnancy
- rheumatism (acute)
- thyroid problems

Medical permission should be sought before treating a client with any of these conditions.

For more information on contraindications see Chapter 5.

You now know what lymphatic drainage massage is and when to use it. The next section explains how it works and the techniques used.

HOW LYMPHATIC DRAINAGE MASSAGE WORKS

Both types of circulation, blood and lymph rely on muscles to act as pumps, particularly in the lower body. All forms of exercise, particularly walking and running help stimulate the circulation by working the muscles and helping the flow of blood and lymph; massage is another form of this stimulation with the added bonus of more focus on areas that need it. When muscles are tired, overworked or damaged they cannot pump as effectively and blood and lymph circulation are therefore not as efficient. This slows down the removal of waste, the distribution of nutrients and oxygen and lowers immunity. At a very simple level this may cause tiredness, swelling and fluid retention. However, in the long term it may cause permanently weakened immunity, congestion of the skin and cells (acne, pimples, cellulite) and lymphoedema.

The techniques of lymphatic drainage massage

Lymphatic drainage massage combines gentle pressure with soft pumping movements in the direction of the lymph nodes. The pressure should never be too heavy because the lymph vessels are superficial and too much pressure is thought to close the valves in the lymph vessels and stop circulation. Softer tissue should be treated with less pressure. All the movements should be carried out slowly. The movements should be performed:

- with light pressure, thus helping rather than forcing the flow of lymph
- in the direction of the heart and the lymph nodes.

Stationary circles technique

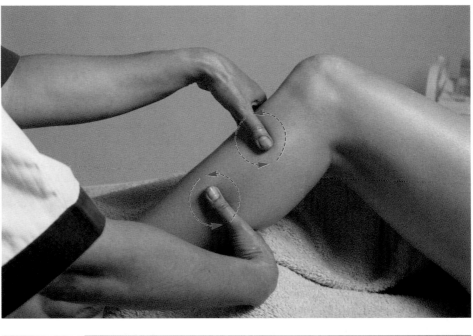

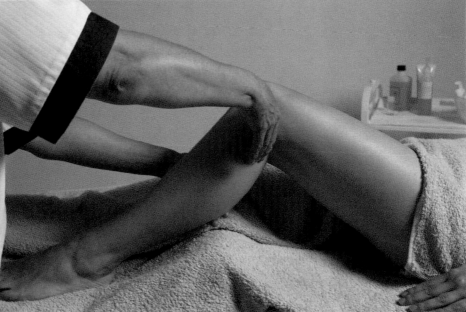

What are the effects of lymphatic drainage massage?

The lymphatic system is a secondary circulation which helps support the blood by collecting and filtering excess tissue fluid from cells. Like all the systems in the body, it has an effect on the others. Therefore, treating it with massage will not only help it function properly but also improve the function of other body systems.

The skin

Skin problems are often caused by inefficient waste removal and the build-up of bacteria. Lymphatic drainage can help eliminate waste and thus decongest the skin, improving its tone and texture and reducing puffiness. The action of massage also encourages desquamation which helps remove dead skin cells, cell regeneration which aids healing and excretion which helps clear toxins from the skin preventing congestion.

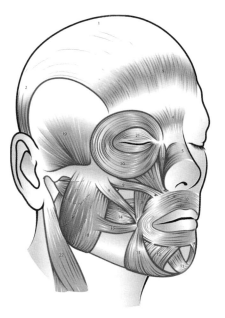

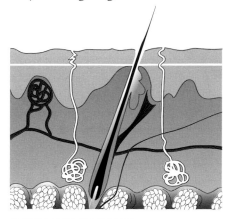

Cross-section of the skin

The muscular system

Waste, particularly lactic acid, prevents muscles from working properly, thus causing them to feel tired, stiff, sore and achy. Lymphatic drainage massage helps speed up the elimination of waste from muscles thus getting rid of the pain and soreness and enabling them to function properly.

The circulatory system

Lymphatic drainage massage helps the lymphatic system to work properly which in turn helps the circulation by removing excess fluid from cells. It is especially important for the removal of excess protein molecules. These are too large to pass through the walls of the venous capillaries and because they retain water they cause fluid retention and bloating. Massaging and promoting lymphatic drainage helps the lymphatic system to collect this excess protein thus helping the circulation to collect any excess water.

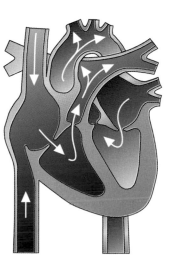

The heart

LYMPHATIC DRAINAGE MASSAGE

CLIENT PROFILE

Ms A is a 45-year-old female who works part-time as an administration assistant. She has noticed a change in her body recently which has been confirmed as the beginning of the menopause. She has begun a programme of exercise on a regular basis, which consists of cardio vascular workout and a gentle weight exercise. She attends the gym 4 to 5 times a week and her diet is good, consisting of all the food groups recommended. Her weight is within the Body Mass Index, although she has cellulite on the buttocks and upper legs.

Treatment plan:

Ms A would like to receive lymphatic drainage massage to aid her cellulite appearance. The agreed plan for treatment would be one massage each week over a three week period. Today the treatment will consist of a full lymphatic drainage massage. She has never received a treatment of lymphatic drainage massage before and therefore it is important that the entire body is treated so the client can experience the whole treatment. All Ms A's expectations were discussed during the consultation, along with the effects and benefits of the treatment.

Client Consultation Form – Lymphatic Drainage Massage

College Name:
College Number:
Student Name:
Student Number:
Date:

Client Name: Ms A
Address: 123, Y street

Profession: Part time Admin Assistant
Tel. No: Day 1234 5678
        Eve 9123 4567

PERSONAL DETAILS

Age group: ☐ Under 20   ☐ 20–30   ☐ 30–40   ☑ 40–50   ☐ 50–60   ☐ 60+
Lifestyle: ☑ Active   ☐ Sedentary
Last visit to the doctor: Around 6 months
GP Address: 456 A Street
No. of children (if applicable): 2 (Grown up)
Date of last period (if applicable): Around 7 days ago

CONTRAINDICATIONS REQUIRING MEDICAL PERMISSION – in circumstances
where medical permission cannot be obtained clients must give their informed consent in writing prior to treatment (select where/if appropriate):

☐ Fever
☐ Contagious or infectious diseases
☐ Under the influence of recreational drugs
    or alcohol
☐ Diarrhoea and vomiting
☐ Residual Malaria
☐ History of TB

☐ Cardiac Insufficiency
☐ Recent Thrombosis
☐ Active Cancer
☐ Medical Oedema
☐ Undiagnosed lumps and bumps
☐ Kidney Infections
☐ Undiagnosed pain

CONTRAINDICTIONS THAT RESTRICT TREATMENT
(select where/if appropriate):

☐ Pregnancy
☐ Cardio vascular conditions (thrombosis, phlebitis,
    hypertension, hypotension, heart conditions)
☐ Any condition already being treated by a GP or
    another complementary practitioner
☐ Medical oedema
☐ Osteoporosis
☐ Arthritis
☐ Nervous/Psychotic conditions
☐ Epilepsy
☐ Recent operations
☐ Diabetes
☐ Asthma
☐ Bells Palsy

☐ Trapped/Pinched nerve
☐ Inflamed nerve
☐ Acute rheumatism
☐ Cancer
☐ Postural deformities
☐ Spastic conditions
☐ Kidney infections
☐ Whiplash
☐ Slipped disc
☐ Undiagnosed pain
☐ When taking prescribed medication
☐ Gastric ulcers
☐ Hernia

LOCALISED CONTRAINDICATIONS

☐ Varicose veins
☐ Bruises
☐ Abrasions
☐ Cuts
☐ Sunburn
☐ Skin diseases

☐ Hormonal implants
☐ Recent fractures (minimum three of months)
☐ After a heavy meal
☐ Abdomen (first few days of menstruation)
☐ Pregnancy (after medical permission has been
    obtained, not on the abdomen

WRITTEN PERMISSION REQUIRED BY:

☐ GP/Specialist   ☐ Informed consent
Either of which should be attached to the consultation form.

LYMPHATIC DRAINAGE MASSAGE

124

PERSONAL INFORMATION (select if/where appropriate):

Muscular/Skeletal problems: ☐ Back ☐ Aches/Pain ☐ Stiff joints ☑ Headaches

Digestive problems: ☐ Constipation ☐ Bloating ☐ Liver/Gall bladder ☐ Stomach

Circulation: ☐ Heart ☐ Blood pressure ☐ Fluid retention ☐ Tired legs ☐ Varicose veins
☑ Cellulite ☐ Kidney problems ☐ Cold hands and feet ☐ Borderline low blood pressure 110/80

Gynaecological: ☐ Irregular periods ☐ P.M.T ☑ Menopause ☐ H.R.T ☐ Pill ☐ Coil

Nervous system: ☐ Migraine ☐ Tension ☐ Stress ☐ Depression

Immune system: ☐ Prone to infections ☐ Sore throats ☐ Colds ☐ Chest ☐ Sinuses

Regular antibiotic/medication taken? ☐ Yes ☑ No

If yes, which ones: ....

Herbal remedies taken? ☐ Yes ☑ No

If yes, which ones: ....

Ability to relax: ☐ Good ☑ Moderate ☐ Poor

Sleep patterns: ☑ Good ☐ Poor ☐ Average No. of hours 8

Do you see natural daylight in your workplace? ☑ Yes ☐ No

Do you work at a computer? ☑ Yes ☐ No If yes how many hours 3

Do you eat regular meals? ☑ Yes ☐ No

Do you eat in a hurry? ☐ Yes ☑ No

Do you take any food/vitamin supplements? ☐ Yes ☑ No

If yes, which ones: ....

How many portions of each of these items does your diet contain per day?

Fresh fruit: 2 Fresh vegetables: 2 Protein: 1 source? Meat

Dairy produce: 1 Sweet things: 1 Added salt: 0 Added sugar: 0

How many units of these drinks do you consume per day?

Tea: 0 Coffee: 1 Fruit juice: 0 Water: 0 Soft drinks: 0 Others: 4

Do you suffer from food allergies? ☐ Yes ☑ No **Bingeing?** ☐ Yes ☑ No **Overeating?** ☐ Yes ☑ No

Do you smoke? ☐ No ☑ Yes How many per day? 1–5

Do you drink alcohol? ☐ No ☑ Yes How many units per day? 1

Do you exercise? ☐ None ☐ Occasional ☐ Irregular ☑ Regular

Types: ....

What is your skin type? ☐ Dry ☐ Oil ☑ Combination ☐ Sensitive ☐ Dehydrated

Do you suffer/have you suffered from: ☐ Dermatitis ☐ Acne ☐ Eczema ☐ Psoriasis
☐ Allergies ☐ Hay Fever ☐ Asthma ☐ Skin cancer

Stress level: 1–10 (10 being the highest)

At work 6 At home 4

Reason for treatment: Ms A would like to experience a new technique of massage. She is also hoping that the massage will aid in detoxification and will have a therapeutic effect aiding the client wellbeing.

....

....

....

....

....

....

....

TREATMENT 1

How the client felt during the treatment:

Ms A found it quite difficult to relax at the beginning of the treatment, this was owing to her anticipation of the forthcoming treatment and her desire to be aware of every detail, including the touch of the massage.

She found the pressure of lymphatic drainage massage very light compared to previous massage techniques that she had received in the past. She eventually began to relax after about 15 minutes and started to close her eyes and begin to settle.

How the client felt after the treatment:

Ms A felt quite relaxed after the massage, however she did not sleep during the massage and was also quite thirsty. I offered the client some water, at room temperature, which she drank. She wanted to rest for a short time before being helped off the couch. I stayed with her until she indicated that she was ready to move.

Home care advice given:

I advised Ms A to be aware of several points.

1. Drink plenty of water to flush out toxins as this will aid in detoxification as this was one of her reasons for the treatment.
2. Keep warm, as this will aid the blood circulation to flow. If the blood circulation continues to flow the lymphatic system will work to remove toxins and waste, again to help one of her reasons for treatment. Cellulite is a condition of stagnation therefore keeping the vascular system working increases the removal of waste.
3. Ms A may suffer a headache after treatment, this is due to the movement of waste and the body dealing with the removal, this is a common after-effect of lymphatic drainage massage and which can be part of the 'healing crisis'.
4. Keeping up with regular exercise and good diet will enhance the treatment.

Reflective practice:

As this was one of my first case studies for lymphatic drainage massage, I had to have my routine notes on hand. The treatment progressed well, even though I had to check my routine notes several times. I am sure with more practice I will remember the routine and that I will feel more professional in my approach. My pressure was not consistent throughout the massage and I believe this was due to the fact that I was checking my notes and not fully focusing. I was well prepared for the treatment and the consultation went well. Ms A appeared to relax as she smiled and gave a small laugh, which indicated positive body language towards me. I am looking forward to seeing her next week and gaining her feedback on the treatment. My aim for the following treatment is to improve the pressure consistency.

Overall conclusion of case study:

The experience of lymphatic drainage massage from Ms A was positive. The technique of lymphatic drainage massage is very light and therefore the client may not feel an instant change in her body. She will hopefully take on board my aftercare advice and drink plenty of water to flush out the toxins. The main purpose of the treatment was to enhance her wellbeing and aid in cellulite reduction. She left the treatment room satisfied and content.

50% OFF! FULL ACCESS

DON'T FORGET NOW YOU CAN USE A RANGE OF ONLINE LEARNING RESOURCES FOR JUST £10 (NORMAL RRP £20)

The Massage e-Learning Resource has been designed to enhance your learning experience

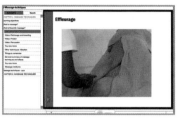

☐ Bring knowledge to life with videos of each technique as well as a full massage routine

☐ Manage your learning with step-by-step modules and integrated 'classroom' sessions

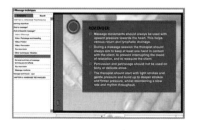

☐ Absorb information on key topics with interactive exercises and learning activities

To login to use these **e-learning resources**, visit **www.emspublishing.co.uk/massage** and follow the onscreen instructions

AN INTRODUCTORY GUIDE TO **Massage**

8 Infant and Child massage

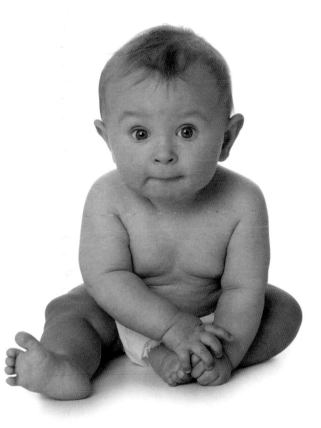

Learning objectives ●

The target knowledge of this chapter is:
- History of infant and child massage
- Benefits of infant and child massage
- Preparing for infant and child massage
- Contraindications to infant and child massage
- Precautions to be taken during infant and child massage
- Techniques of infant and child massage
- Home care

In Brief

Infant and Child Massage is an holistic approach to infant health and child rearing. It combines the tender touch of a nurturer with specific movements and techniques designed to improve the health of any child, from infant and beyond.

HISTORY OF BABY MASSAGE

Baby massage has a very long history and has been a part of eastern cultures for thousands of years – although it has only relatively recently become practised in the west. In eastern cultures massage is part of the daily routine, whereby the grandmother will pass down her skills and knowledge to the new mother. Massage is thought to relax the baby, improve flexibility and protect the skin.

Eastern cultures recognise the importance of body and skin contact as a natural daily custom. Many mothers in such countries as India, Africa and Asia carry out their daily chores with their babies in a sling; enabling the baby to be close to their mother's body and experience her rhythm and movement. This in turn helps to stimulate the baby's emotional and motor development.

WHAT ARE THE BENEFITS?

What are the benefits?

Touch helps the baby and infant to feel loved, safe and secure, which is paramount for self-confidence and personal development. Massage also encourages bonding between the parent and baby to develop which is often neglected in the 21st century as the pace of life becomes ever more demanding. Lack of bonding between parent and child is a factor that could result in psychological and emotional problems throughout the child's development. Babies can be massaged from the first week of birth using only very light effleurage movements, taking care to avoid the abdomen whilst the umbilical cord is healing. After approximately 6 weeks, a light massage may be performed safely which will give the baby a wonderful feeling of wellbeing, security and love – encouraging the baby to thrive.

Infant and Child Massage can include the following benefits:

- Relaxation
- Improved sleep patterns
- Reduced discomfort
- Aiding respiratory problems
- Aiding immune problems
- Enhanced feelings of security
- Increased bonding between infant and
- parent

Apart from the direct benefits for the infant there are also extremely positive aspects for the parent who is performing the massage. These might include some or all of the following:-

- Helps post-natal depression
- Helps with feelings of guilt
- Encouraging relaxation
- Good for 'redundant fathers' mainly due to breastfeeding

Why use Baby Massage?

Many new mothers and fathers find it very difficult to adapt to the demands of a new baby. The crying, sleepless nights and the change of a familiar routine can cause a feeling of helplessness in the parent/guardian and therefore bonding with a newborn is not always a natural consequence and may be a process that needs to be worked on. Once a massage routine has been established it can promote feelings of security, confidence and contentment for both the parent and baby.

You now know where baby massage comes from and the benefits of why it can be used.

PREPARING FOR MASSAGE

Preparing for any type of massage is important but it is particularly so for infants and children. It is of paramount importance that the room, lighting and atmosphere is as relaxing as possible. Both the infant/child and the parent/guardian should be relaxed and comfortable. The baby should never be woken to have a massage and should not be hungry or need changing.

Infants often show signs to indicate that they are ready for interaction and it is invaluable for the therapist to be able to recognise these signs:

- Eyes may widen and face may brighten
- Seeking eye contact
- Hands open with fingers relaxed
- Giggling, babbling or talking
- Smiling

The following points need to be taken into consideration to enable the infant or child and the parent to gain full potential from the massage:-

- Decide where the massage is going to take place – on a couch, floor, lap or bed. Ensure that the area is safe and clean
- The temperature of the room is important for the baby to be relaxed and needs to be roughly 10 degrees above normal, particularly when massaging babies as they lose their body heat more quickly than adults
- Ensure there are no draughts
- Avoid bright or glaring lights
- Play some soft relaxing music
- A few soft toys in case the baby becomes distracted during the massage
- Allow plenty of time
- Soft towels or a small blanket to keep the infant warm and cosy
- Oil or cream
- Tissues and/or wipes

WHEN SHOULDN'T YOU PERFORM A MASSAGE ON YOUR INFANT/CHILD?

Massage is non-invasive, relaxing and natural. It is therefore generally considered a safe treatment for most infants and children. Contraindications are listed to enable the therapist to have a better understanding of the infant/child's condition so as to prevent any harm or discomfort, and to know how to carry out the massage safely.

Contraindications requiring medical referral, or the parent/guardian to indemnify their condition in writing prior to the treatment

- Recent operation/surgery
- Congenital heart condition
- Congenital dislocation of the hip
- Spastic conditions

- Dysfunction of the nervous system
- Epilepsy
- Asthma

Contraindications that restrict treatment

- Fever
- Contagious or infectious diseases
- Recent fractures, sprains and swelling
- Recent haemorrhage
- Jaundice
- Meningitis
- Childhood leukaemia
- Osteoporosis/brittle bones
- Diarrhoea and vomiting
- Recent immunisation (minimum 48 hours)
- Skin disorders

- Inflammatory skin conditions
- Skin allergies
- Cuts and bruises
- Unhealed navel
- Infantile seborrhoeic dermatitis (cradle cap)

It is important to carry out a consultation with the parent/guardian to ensure the infant/child is suitable for massage, and to advise the parent/guardian to seek medical advice if the infant/child is under medical care. It is also important to act in a co-operative manner with other health care professionals and refer cases outside your skill range or therapeutic knowledge to those with relevant qualifications. In addition you should respect the religious, spiritual, social and political views of the parents/guardians and never abuse the relationship between yourself and the parent/guardian or infant/child.

AREAS REQUIRING CAUTION

There are certain areas when massaging babies and small children that require extra care and caution, as pressure over the area may cause damage to underlying structures and/or may cause discomfort.

The areas that require extra care when massaging are as follows:-

- Front of the neck and throat
- Orbital area
- Back of neck
- Spine
- Axilla
- Front and back of elbow
- Brachial region (upper arm)
- Upper lumber (over kidney area)
- Umbilical area
- Femoral triangle
- Popliteal fossa
- Inguinal area

How to do it

Massaging an infant/child is very different to massaging an adult. There are many areas that the therapist/parent/guardian needs to be particularly aware of in order to adapt the pressure and movements accordingly. Always warm the hands prior to massage. This is important when massaging adults, but imperative with infants and children as starting to massage with cold hands could startle them, unsettle them and/or make them cry. Talking to and making eye contact with the infant/child relaxes them making them more receptive to the massage, especially at the beginning of the treatment. Watch out for any arm movements going in and out from the chest as this usually indicates that you should stop the massage because the infant is becoming agitated.

TECHNIQUES OF INFANT AND CHILD MASSAGE

If the infant is quite tiny and has not been massaged before, it might be a good idea to start with just a 5 minute massage so the infant can get use to the feel of the movements. If the infant/child feels uncomfortable having his or her clothes removed, the massage movements can be performed over soft clothing such as a sleep suit (the use of oils or cream are not always necessary).

Starting the massage can be done with the infant lying on their back and massaging the chest or the front of their legs using effleurage.

Effleurage

Effleurage is a gentle, sweeping and relaxing stroke which is used at the beginning and end of a massage and also as a linking movement; this technique will gently increase the circulation of the infant/child. It is often just the fingers in baby massage that maintain contact during the massage, rather than the whole palm of the hand, due to the small surface area being massaged. Hands may also be used simultaneously on larger areas such as the back with the use of thumbs and fingers on the smaller areas. Light pressure is all that should be initially applied, gradually proceeding to a medium or firmer pressure once the infant/child has become familiar with the massage or has increased in size. This movement is the main technique used in infant massage.

Petrissage

This movement produces a kneading action which squeezes and manipulates the tissues using the fingers and thumbs. When massaging an adult this is quite a deep movement and although with an

infant/child it can be quite a firm movement, great care must be taken not to twist the tissue too much or pinch the skin. Depending on the area being massaged, petrissage can be performed with one hand or both. Pressure should be smooth and firm yet still creating a relaxing effect. This in turn will help to release the tension in the infant's muscles and eliminate waste products from the tissues. It is important to ascertain the infant's tissue density before commencing this particular massage movement to help determine the pressure to be used.

Friction

When performing a friction movement within an adult massage it tends to be particularly deep and stimulating. Circular friction movements can still be used for an infant/child massage but the pressure must be considerably lighter. This movement, like petrissage, will help to release tension in the muscles and increase circulation.

HOMECARE

Homecare is an important part of the massage as it helps both the infant/child and the parent/guardian to look after themselves in between massage treatments and to put into practice the advice that the therapist has given. This could include all or any of the following:-
- Healthy eating
- Plenty of fluids
- Fresh air for both parent/guardian and infant/child
- Avoid direct sunlight particularly immediately after massage
- Ensure the infant/child is kept warm again, particularly after the massage as they will have increased circulation and may therefore feel the cold more.
- Allow the infant/child to sleep or relax after the massage

- Monitor the infant/child's response to the massage

After the massage the parent/guardian may notice some differences with the infant/child which should be discussed to alleviate any worries. Any of the following changes are quite normal and should not be cause for concern.
- Increased micturation
- Increased defecation
- Altered feeding patterns
- Altered sleeping patterns
- Contentment

You now know what infant and child massage is, the benefits for both the infant/child and the parent/guardian and the techniques.

INFANT AND CHILD MASSAGE

THE MASSAGE

Massaging the Baby can begin as soon as the mother feels up to it. Firmer, deeper strokes can be applied when the baby is one month old.

Work gently, slowly and softly.

Talk quietly to the baby and maintain eye contact. Heed the baby's responses, they are his/her words. If the baby appears to be responding favourably to a specific stroke, repeat it.

Begin the infant massage with the baby lying on their back on a towel or sheet in front of you.

Ensure the room is warm and comfortable and that your hands are warm too

It is best to choose a light, organic, cold-pressed vegetable oil.

Begin by talking to the baby and letting the baby know you are about to massage them.

Start at the feet and apply sufficient lubrication to allow your hands to "glide", but not "slip". (See below)

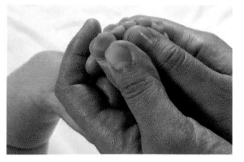

Work your way up the leg paying particular attention to support the knee and work deep into the thigh area.

When both legs are done perform a hip stretch.

Continue to work into the abdominal region and carry out gentle effleurage strokes on the tummy draining into the inguinals. (See photo below)

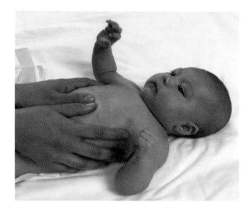

Work on the chest using long fluid strokes across the sternum and out onto the arms, include an arm stretch. (See below)

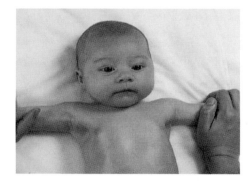

Massage the hands with deliberate strokes working into the fingers. (see below)

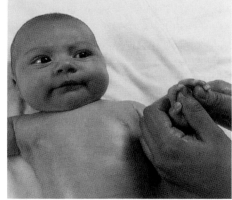

Work up onto the face and use secure strokes on the face using the thumbs. (See below)

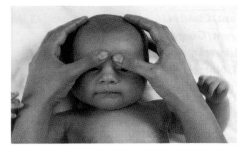

Turn the baby over to work the back and into the bottom. Using strong deliberate strokes up the spine and into the shoulders. (See below)

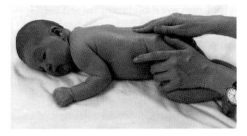

Turn the baby back over and perform a series of connecting strokes from the feet to the head.

Typically these initial massages should take approximately 10 minutes, performed on a daily basis.

As the baby grows the massages can become longer, lasting up to half an hour, carried out three times a week, or as often as you and your baby would like.

Enjoy these special times with the baby and never loose an opportunity to re-enforce positive touch.

INFANT/CHILD PROFILE:

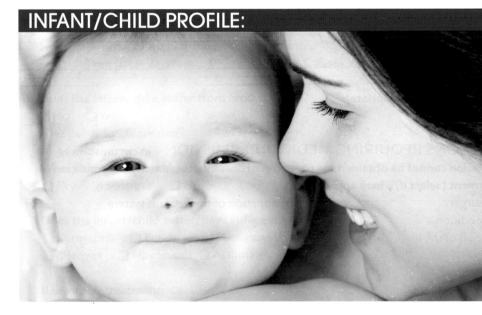

Maisy is a very happy and content little baby girl with lots of smiles. She was born by an emergency c-section after natural labour did not progress as Mrs L's cervix did not dilate. She took to the breast immediately and has been "Feeding for England" ever since.
Maisy is now 3 months old and Mrs L is determined to give her daughter the best start by following the current health authority recommendations that babies do better if fed exclusively by breast for the first 6 months.
Mrs L has tried to express milk to enable her to share feeding times with her husband but finds expressing uncomfortable and, as Maisy feeds so well, she tries to nap when the baby does or she gets "unbearably tired".

TREATMENT 1

Details of how the therapist conducted the treatment:

Maisy had fallen asleep during the consultation and, whilst I demonstrated the massage sequence on a baby doll, Maisy woke from her nap and I repeated the movements for Mrs L to copy on Maisy.

I pointed out all the areas that needed to be avoided, taking care to explain why, and to invite questions from Mrs L. Mrs L was able to copy the movements well.

Details of how the infant/child reacted during and after the treatment:

Maisy napped throughout the the entire demonstration, she was so content we did not want to disturb her.

Mrs L did very well with the movements on Maisy when she woke up. Maisy seemed quite content during the massage until Mrs L worked on her back. This could be because it was her first massage and she was unsure of what was going on.

Maisy gurgled happily whilst Mrs L got her dressed; she seems a very happy and settled baby.

Details of home care advice given:

I gave Mrs L leaflets to remind her on the areas to avoid and how to prepare both herself and Maisy for their massage sessions at home. I also gave her some apricot kernel oil to use during the massage.

I encouraged Mrs L to continue to rest when Maisy does to help keep her energy levels up and reminded her to nourish herself well and drink plenty of water as she continues to breastfeed. I also gently suggested she have a chat to her health visitor about her tiredness and said she may like to try a massage herself sometime.

Overall conclusion of the case study including reflective practice:

It was lovely that Maisy was so content after the treatment; I'm sure both Mother and baby will enjoy experiencing the massage at home.

I think it was useful to demonstrate on the doll first. Mrs L seemed to be able to follow the movements well on Maisy when she woke up.

Mrs L was very attentive but it was clear that she was so very tired. I'm glad I had prepared leaflets as I'm sure she wasn't able to take in all I said.

I hope she has a chat with her health visitor as I suggested; she seemed to become almost tearful when she spoke about her "unbearable tiredness". I'll check during their next appointment.

Mrs L did very well with the movements and I'm sure she'll get on well with massaging Maisy.

TREATMENT 2

Details of how the therapist conducted the treatment:

As Maisy was awake during this session it was lovely to observe Mrs L using the movements I showed her last time so well.

Everything started off fine, but as soon as Maisy was turned on to her front she was less happy. Mrs L seemed to get quite upset that she was doing something wrong and told me that she'd not been able to finish the massage at home at all yet. I reassured her that she was doing fine and that some babies just aren't all that happy on their tummies. I encouraged Mrs L to pick Maisy up to comfort her and, as soon as she did, Maisy was all smiles again. I remarked that she was obviously much happier this way and showed them a different back sequence technique on my demonstration doll in the upright position.

Mrs L copied the movments on Maisy and was able to complete the massage; she was delighted that it wasn't something that she was doing wrong.

Details of how the infant/child reacted during and after the treatment:

Maisy was bright and alert during this session. She gurgled and giggled during the first part of the massage and particularly seemed to like her feet being worked on. She also responded immediately to Mrs L's voice.

It was clear they both enjoyed the massage until Maisy was turned on to her front which she clearly did not like as she squirmed, wriggled and arched her back, squealing and straining to try and look round at her Mother.

As soon as Mrs L picked Maisy up she gurgled happily again and seemed to enjoy the rest of the massage being performed in this position.

Details of home care advice given:

I congratulated Mrs L on her massage technique and said I was impressed how quickly she'd picked up the movements. She remarked that she had really enjoyed massaging Maisy until "the back bit" and was delighted I'd shown her an alternative way of doing the back.

I remarked to Mrs L that she seemed a little brighter this time and not quite so tired and she told me that she'd taken my advice and spoken to her health visitor who'd suggested cutting out the 2am feed. Apparently, after 2 nights of realising that all she was going to get for waking up at 2am was Daddy with some water, Maisy had not bothered since and now sleeps from 7pm to 7am!

As Maisy liked her feet being touched so much I gave Mrs L a leaflet on baby Reflexology which she may like to try.

OVERALL CONCLUSION INCLUDING REFLECTIVE PRACTICE ●

It's so lovely to see both Mother and baby benefit from massage. I'm glad I was able to show them another way of working on the back as it obviously suited Maisy much better.

I was also pleased that Mrs L had taken my advice and spoken to her health visitor about her tiredness and also that I'd thought to suggest it to her.

50% OFF
FULL ACCESS

DON'T FORGET NOW YOU CAN USE A RANGE OF ONLINE LEARNING RESOURCES FOR JUST £10 (NORMAL RRP £20)

The Massage e-Learning Resource has been designed to enhance your learning experience

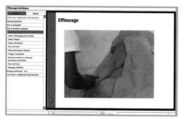

☐ Bring knowledge to life with videos of each technique as well as a full massage routine

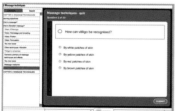

☐ Manage your learning with step-by-step modules and integrated 'classroom' sessions

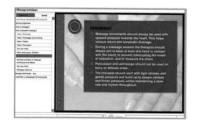

☐ Absorb information on key topics with interactive exercises and learning activities

To login to use these **e-learning resources**, visit **www.emspublishing.co.uk/massage** and follow the onscreen instructions

AN INTRODUCTORY GUIDE TO
Massage

9 Stone Therapy Massage

Learning objectives

The target knowledge of this chapter is:
- History of Stone Therapy Massage (and its various concepts)
- Benefits of Stone Therapy Massage
- Techniques of Stone Therapy Massage
- Definition of the Chakras & the Aura
- Carrying out a treatment

In Brief

Stone Therapy Massage combines the use of hot and cold stones with traditional massage techniques to bring about deep relaxation and homeostasis on a physical, psychological and spiritual level. This modern day treatment draws upon ancient healing arts and traditions to deliver a deeper massage with less exertion required from the therapist.

THE HISTORY OF STONE THERAPY MASSAGE AND ITS VARIOUS CONCEPTS

Stone Therapy Massage or Geothermotherapy (geo meaning Earth, thermotherapy relating to the alternate use of hot and cold) is really an extension of manual massage the history of which you will already have learnt (see chapter 1).

Like massage, the use of stones in ceremonial rituals, for spiritual or indeed medicinal purposes, dates back thousands of years spanning many civilizations. Man's fascination with linking specific types of stone for certain purposes is clearly reflected in formations such as the stone circles at Stonehenge and Avebury – erected approximately 4500 years ago, and in the Egyptian Pyramids.

Who used Stones?

In China the application of heated stones to relieve tired aching muscles dates back over 3000 years.

The Incas built large temples in which to worship, having first coated their stones in gold.

The Hawaiian Kahunas (priests or elders) used massage with warm lava stones wrapped in the moist bark of the Noni plant, thought to restore a person's life force – the practice of which is still in use today.

The Russians traditionally used heated black stones (renowned for their warming release of energy) in their baths. The many tribes of Native American Indians used stones (affectionately referring to them as the 'Stone Clan People') for reasons ranging from pure warmth, to rites and initiation ceremonies. Their beliefs in the provision of Mother Earth and Father Sky, as well as honouring the forces of nature and respecting the five basic elements of

water, wood, fire, earth and metal, are all integral concepts in the theories upon which treatment is based in the present day.

Which stones are used?

Pumice stone, a volcanic rock, is used in nail products to 'buff out' ridges and as an exfoliant for rough, dry skin, the world over.

Crystal, a term which is derived from the Ancient Greek term 'Krystallos' meaning 'ice', or semi precious gem stones have been used throughout history for healing, personal reflection and meditation, as well as for ornamental purposes. Abundant in Egyptian tombs and referred to in Greek mythology, crystals were used by Native Indians and Aztecs and Mayans, who used them in ceremonies and rituals. Crystals work to help balance the body's natural rhythm and when applied on, or near to, an area their individual vibrational frequency can help to correct any imbalance in the corresponding Chakra (see below).

Auras

All living things have an electro magnetic field around them called the 'Aura' (see below). Few people are able to see this without practise, but it can be felt; when a person enters a room we can sometimes 'feel' their presence before we see them, at other times we may feel 'tension in the air', having walked into a room where people have been arguing. Historically, artists would paint halos around the heads of spiritual people. Biblically, writers would refer to 'rays of light' emanating from around angels, men and women. Terms used today such as 'pea green with envy', 'feeling blue', 'angry red' and 'radiant beauty' are all said to be reflections upon how a person's emotions and mood may affect the colour of their aura at that particular time.

Kirlian photography is said to be able to capture the colour and size of a person's electromagnetic field, but this has not been scientifically proven.

THE DEVELOPMENT OF STONE THERAPY

The use of hot and cold water for therapeutic effects is referred to as 'Hydrotherapy' an example of which would be heated baths and cold plunge pools. Its uses have been recorded as early as the Ancient Egyptians whose Royalty bathed in essential oils and flowers. The Romans had communal public baths and Hippocrates, the Greek 'Father of Medicine' prescribed bathing in spring water to help sickness.

The Kneipp Theory

Sebastian Kneipp, born in the Bavarian region of Germany in 1821, was a great advocate of Hydrotherapy and a founder of the Naturopathic Medicine movement. His methods of healing rested upon five main doctrines – hydrotherapy, herbalism, exercise, nutrition and spirituality. He has had a great influence upon the development of the Spa industry, as it is today, having invented the 'sitz' bath and through his 'Kneipp Cure' form of hydrotherapy. The active agents in these treatments however, are the use of heat and cold – water is merely the method of application. The application of heat and

cold is known as the term 'Thermotherapy' and in the case of Stone Massage, it is the use of stones, both hot and cold, which act as a natural stimulus, having a dramatic effect upon the systems of the body.

Stone Massage

There are many forms of Stone Massage available today, but it is Mary Nelson who must be acknowledged as the pioneer of these treatments. Coming from Tucson, Arizona in the USA, she first began her work upon the various aspects of this treatment in the early 1970s. She continued to practise and build upon all facets of her routine whilst researching the various theories (outlined above) and incorporating them into her treatments. In 1993, the culmination of these concepts led to 'the birth' of Stone Therapy. It is to Nelson that we must accredit the various techniques upon which the current stone massage routines are based. It was her who was inspired to use stones as a massage tool and combine all of the factors into what we now know to be Stone Therapy Massage, or Geothermotherapy.

BENEFITS AND TECHNIQUES OF STONE THERAPY MASSAGE

What is Stone Therapy Massage?

Based upon traditional Swedish massage techniques, hot and cold stones are used to massage the client. The stones may also be placed in strategic positions on top and beneath the body, to create a therapeutic and holistic effect. This will benefit both the area concerned and the person in general. In addition to the

stones, crystals may also be incorporated to the treatment, as they too will have a 'balancing' effect upon the client, helping to achieve total homeostasis. A full body treatment can take anything up to 90 minutes and, as with massage, is generally carried out with the client undressed.

A successful treatment may still be

TOWER HAMLETS COLLEGE
POPLAR HIGH STREET
LONDON
E14 0AF

STONE THERAPY

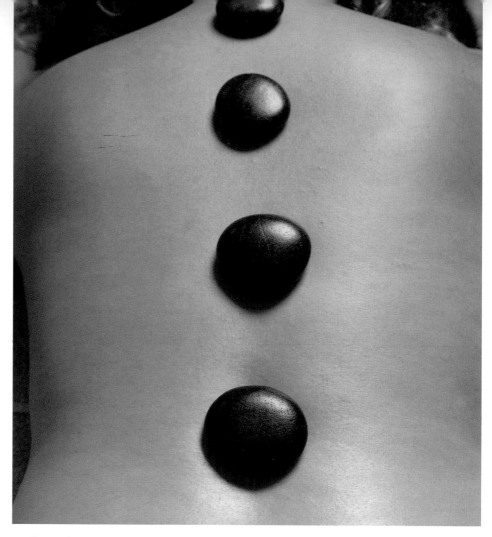

performed over the client's clothes, but the temperature of the stones must be higher than normal to accommodate this.

Hot or cold stones may be effectively incorporated into many other therapies, enhancing the treatments furthermore. An example would be in an Indian Head Massage routine (see chapter 10) using the hot stones to massage the back and cold stones for pressure point work on the face.

What type of stones should be used for the treatment?

Basalt is the recommended stone for a hot stone treatment. It is the most common of igneous rocks (igneous, meaning that they formed from molten lava) and there are several varieties, all of which have an excellent capacity to retain heat. The stones can be found in any area of the world known for volcanic activity such as, Tenerife, Italy, Japan and Indonesia. Their colour is generally grey or black, being rich in minerals such as iron and magnesium, and the presence of other minerals such as olivine, may give a green appearance to the stones. Registering at seven on the Moh's scale of hardness, they are dense and quite durable.

Marble is an ideal stone to use in conjunction with, and as a contrast to, Basalt. It is a sedimentary rock sourced mainly from the ocean. These rocks are generally formed by compression of a combination of marine or plant life, calcite and limestone and other rock particles. Over thousands or even millions of years, weight from overlying sediments condenses the various lower layers together to form a compact mass. Marble rocks, rank at three on the Moh's scale of hardness and, as such, are quite easily scratched. Generally white in appearance, there can be possible colour variations, or 'veins,' depending upon any additional components, like sand or clay, that have been compressed into the rock formation. These stones are renowned for their 'cool' energies. Stones shaped from the crystal Jade are beneficial for use in the treatment as they can be used for both hot and cool applications. However, the purchase price for these kits is usually much more expensive than their Basalt and Marble counterparts.

What Massage Medium is used?

Generally, the preferred massage medium is oil, as this will help the stones to retain their heat and lubricate the area being treated. (See chapter 10 for the various carrier oils.) The properties of the chosen oil may also bring benefits to the specific skin type and the heat will aid its absorption. Creams and other products may be used, such as anti-cellulite creams and firming serums, as long as they remain stable when exposed to heat. The use of essential oils, by a qualified Aromatherapist, can also give an added dimension to the treatment (see chapter 12).

What are the benefits of using hot stones?

- One stroke with a hot Basalt stone is thought to be the equivalent to ten manual massage strokes, so results are achieved more quickly and efficiently. Care must be taken however, not to over treat an area.
- The stones allow for deeper penetration of pressure and work upon an area, without tiring the therapist and causing undue stress on wrists and joints.

- The heat from the stones will permeate through the client's body causing vasodilation to occur. This will bring more oxygen and nutrients to the tissues and speed up the removal of carbon dioxide and waste.
- Tired aching muscles will be restored to their normal state more readily, as lactic acid elimination is increased.
- The lymphatic system will be stimulated, increasing its circulation, and thereby aiding the detoxification processes.
- Cell metabolism (microcirculation) is increased, aiding cell functioning and the healing repair of tissues.
- Body metabolism is increased, improving the efficiency of the body systems in general.
- A state of deep relaxation occurs, as the warmth from the stones soothes nerve endings.
- The stones absorb negative energies from the client, whilst acting as a barrier to protect the therapist.

What are the benefits of using cold stones?

These work in complete contrast to the heated stones, bringing about the opposite physiological effects.

- Vasoconstriction narrows blood vessels, reducing the blood supply and microcirculation to the area. This will therefore cool and soothe any areas of inflammation, as well as reducing fluid retention.
- An analgesic effect takes place so a numbing or reduction of sensitivity in the area will occur. Under the correct circumstances, this again allows for deeper work upon the body.
- The change in temperature by the application of cold stones makes for a sharp intake of breath, improving the oxygenation of blood. (Good client care means that the client should

always be warned before the initial application of the cold stones).

- Used on the body, cold stones can help unblock congested areas. When used on the face, it helps to decongest the sinuses, whilst placement over the eyes can help reduce dark circles.
- The tightening and firming impact that cold has on the skin means that flesh will be firmed and a toning effect will occur. This is something that is desirable to clients, whether it is face, or body.

The alternate application of hot and cold will have a much greater effect, than when used individually.

What are the psychological benefits of using the stones?

- A treatment can bring about feelings of spiritual calmness and/or mental invigoration.
- Feelings of contentment and wellbeing, pampering and warmth.
- The vibrational energy of the stones resonates with those of the chakras

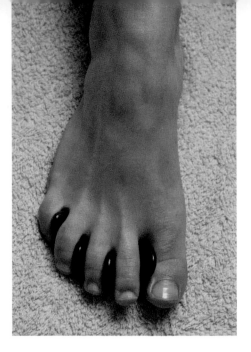

and balance is restored; hopefully attaining total homeostasis on a physical, psychological and spiritual level, although a client may require several treatments in order to achieve this.

You now know the history of Stone Therapy and its uses, and the benefits of using Geothermotherapy for the body and mind.

WHAT IS THE CHAKRA?

'Chakra' is the Sanskrit word for 'wheel of light', the philosophy of which originates from India. Chakras are viewed as 'spinning lights of energy' or 'vortexes'. Although it is thought that there are many minor chakras throughout the body (e.g. the soles of the feet, palms of hands, backs of knees) there are seven main chakras: the root or base ('Muladhara') facing downwards; sacral ('Svadhisthana'); solar plexus ('Manipura'); heart ('Anahata'); throat ('Vishudda'); third eye ('Ajna'); all lying horizontally to the body; and the crown chakra ('Sahasrara') facing upwards. These energy centres are positioned in front of the spinal column and aligned vertically up the spine. Opening directly into the auric field, they link the physical,

mental, emotional and spiritual functions. Each one is associated with specific body glands or organs and can be depicted by a particular colour: root (red), sacral (orange), solar plexus (yellow), heart (green or pink), throat (turquoise), third eye (indigo), crown (violet or white).

How does treatment help Chakras?

The state of health of each chakra can affect the corresponding body part. All are of equal importance and if one is spinning too quickly, or slowly, it will have a domino effect upon the others, causing imbalance and potential illness. They are linked to the physical body by the endocrine system and open into and

Chakra Chart

Chakra Name	Associated Colour	Purpose & Related Body Area	Associated Gemstone /Crystal	Possible Imbalances
Root/Base	Red	Our grounding energy centre. Covers sexual vitality & reproductive organs.	Garnet or Bloodstone	Problems in the hips, legs, lower back & sexual organs.
Sacral	Orange	Relationships and social interactions with others. Responsible for lower intestines & digestive system.	Orange jasper or carnelian	Kidney weakness, stiff lower back, constipation and related muscle spasms, skin irritations.
Solar Plexus	Yellow	Emotional balance. Responsible for pancreas, stomach and liver area.	Tigers Eye or Citrine	Digestive & liver problems, diabetes, nervous exhaustion, insomnia and food allergies.
Heart	Green/Pink	Love centre, controls unconditional feeling and thoughts. Responsible for the heart, thymus gland, circulatory and respiratory systems.	Rose quartz or green jade	Heart attack, high blood pressure, circulatory problems, difficulty breathing and loneliness.
Throat	Turquoise	Encourages communication. Responsible for vocal cords, thyroid glands and parathyroid glands.	Turquoise or aquamarine.	Hyper/hypothyroid, sore throat, laryngitis, inflammation and neck pain.
Third Eye/Brow	Indigo	The psychic energy centre- this chakra governs our senses. Responsible for pituitary gland, face, eyes, nose and sinuses.	Sodalite or lapis lazuli	Headaches, blurred vision, blindness and eyestrain. Mental health problems. Muscle spasms in the shoulder and neck area.
Crown	Violet/white	Spiritual gateway. Our higher self. Responsible for the pineal gland, our skull and brain.	Amethyst or clear crystal quartz.	Migraine, stress, headaches & depression. Also scalp problems.

exist within the 'auric field' (see below). This means that the auric field is directly linked to the activity of the chakras. When treating a person, the transmission of energy can help to clear both the chakras and the aura, rebalancing and re-energising a person and having an uplifting effect upon their mood.

What is the Aura?

The aura, originating from the Greek word for 'breeze', is an egg shaped three-dimensional electromagnetic field, which surrounds the body, extending by anything up to four feet. Changes In a person's physical or mental health, spiritual or emotional wellbeing, can affect the size, shape and colour of the aura. The first three layers are, from closest to the body outwards: the etheric body (linked to the base chakra), emotional body (linked to the sacral chakra), mental body (linked to the solar plexus chakra), astral body (linked to the heart chakra), etheric template (linked to the throat chakra), celestial body (linked to the third eye chakra) and the ketheric body (linked to the crown chakra). The first three are thought to be linked with the physical plane, while the last three are thought to be linked to the spiritual plane.

How can treatment help the aura?

Whenever we touch someone we are working with energy and, as such, can have an effect upon their 'auric field'. In channelling this Universal Energy (known as 'Chi' in China, Ki in Japan, Prana in India) through the client, as we perform a massage treatment, we can help to clear meridians (energy channels running through the body), the chakras and the aura. If the chakras and energy field are out of balance, so too will be the body.

What are the benefits of incorporating crystals into a treatment?

When crystals are incorporated into a treatment there is an added dimension, relating to the balancing of the chakras and overall energy of the person, which is present. The addition will further aid the stones in their aim to 'emotionally balance,' encouraging the client to feel more positive in their outlook, or help moderate any dominant characteristics.

Which crystals should be used?

Crystal therapy is an interesting and vast subject matter in that all crystals possess individual healing powers. Some, however, are more suited to work with certain chakras than others. Generally

speaking the opaque, more densely coloured crystals will resonate to balance the lower chakras more effectively. The more translucent or transparent crystals, resonate at a higher frequency to balance the higher chakras. Whilst qualified crystal therapists may wish to draw upon their knowledge and incorporate specific gem stones to address particular problem areas, for the purpose of a stone massage treatment and the remit of this book, the following choice of gemstones have been suggested. The following are considered to be predominantly suited to the areas or chakra concerned:

- Base or root chakra - use garnet, agate or bloodstone
- Sacral - use carnelian, moonstone or orange jasper
- Solar plexus - use tiger's eye, yellow citrine or amber
- Heart - use rose quartz, green jade or tourmaline
- Throat - use lapis lazuli, turquoise or aquamarine
- Third eye or brow chakra - use purple fluorite, sodalite or opal
- Crown - use amethyst, clear crystal quartz or white topaz

It is not by coincidence that the colours of the chosen crystals are in keeping with those of their associate chakras. Indeed, the correlation between the two increases the effectiveness.

How do I do it?

The same techniques used for Swedish Massage (see chapter 3) are utilised and simulated in Stone Massage. The difference is that a stone sits between the therapist's hand and the client. All of the benefits (see chapter 4) of a particular movement are achieved more quickly, with fewer strokes. It is not advisable to perform tapotement with the stones, as the style of these movements makes this totally impractical. Hot stones may be used with each of the massage techniques described below, as can cold. However, the use of cold stones is particularly beneficial over areas of inflammation, for performing frictions, cross fibre frictions and trigger point work.

What precautionary measures need to be taken?

- Give the client a glass of water to drink prior to the treatment – ideally when carrying out the consultation for prevention against dehydration and help with the detoxification process.
- Always carry out a thermal safety test prior to treatment
- Always check the temperature of the stones with the thermometer prior to use.
- Always wear gloves to remove hot stones from the heater.
- If the stones feel too hot/cold to the therapist, never apply them to the client. If so, turn the stones in the hands until a comfortable temperature is reached, or dip in cool water.
- Ensure that the client has had a light meal prior to the treatment. They should be neither hungry, nor full from a heavy meal.
- Once in contact with the skin, keep hot stones moving.
- Always ensure that a towel or layer of cloth is placed between skin and hot stationary stone.
- Care should be taken when working over bony areas and never catch bony prominences e.g. the knee.
- Prolonged use of cold stones over the kidney region, or any unisolated area, is unwise as the 'chill factor' could lead to problems with the urinary system.

- Check that the pressure is comfortable, as use of the stones provides a deeper massage.

With each of the following movements, the alternate application of heat and cold should be considered and the respective stones used accordingly.

Effleurage
(Refer to chapter 3 for explanation of traditional massage techniques and chapter 4 for their individual benefits) Start with manual effleurage movements to spread the medium and introduce your hands to the client/area. Remove two stones from the heater and where necessary, turn in the hands to absorb heat and give a light coverage of massage medium. The backs of the hands should be placed onto the area to be worked for a couple of seconds then turn the hands over and commence the effleurage stroke. The stones should sit comfortably in the palms of the hand as they travel over the skin. The fingers should not grip the stones, but work as one, contouring to the area being treated. Just as with

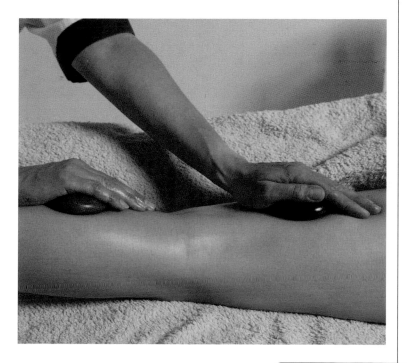

normal effleurage, pressure should always be toward the heart and contact with the client should not be broken until the movement has been completed. Do not worry if the stones 'flip over' whilst carrying out the movement – fresh warmth will be delivered to the tissues, the first time that this happens. The flat surface of the stone is generally used for these movements.

Petrissage

The flat surface of the stones (as described above) may be used in conjunction with palmar kneading, but more pressure is applied. Wringing and picking up are again performed with the stone nestled in the hand. Fingers and thumbs lift and manipulate the flesh in a rhythmical fashion as usual, but the flat of the stone is pressed into the body on

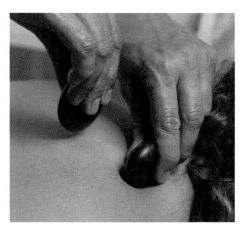

Petrissage – alternate kneading

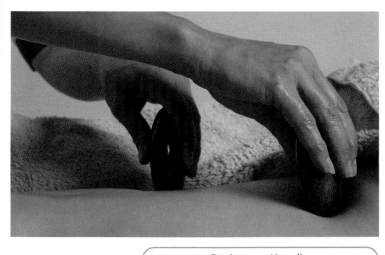

the downward movement by the palm of the hand. Continue with the movement until the whole area or muscle has been covered.

Remember: these movements should only be carried out after effleurage has been performed.

Frictions

The edges/sides of the stones are ideal replacements to the use of fingers and thumbs in this movement. Deeper pressure may be applied effortlessly and the addition of heat from the stone will render the muscle more receptive to further work, more quickly. Holding the stone as one would an eraser, work back and forth along the knotted fibres of the muscle. Imagine that areas of tension are being 'rubbed out'. Again, ensure that the area has been previously worked upon with effleurage and petrissage movements prior to commencing work. This method of application may be used with chilled stones where there are areas of inflammation, but always be guided by client response; if the client expresses pain then stop immediately.

Cross Fibre Frictions

Having worked along the muscle fibre (as above), apply pressure working across the fibres. This will help to break down adhesions lining the muscle fibres and between the muscles and the skin (this is a good technique to use against stubborn cellulite). Chilled stones are ideal for this movement.

Tapotement

These movements may be incorporated into the routine if desired, but not with the use of the stones. The compounded effects of the temperature of the hot and cold stones, their vibrational energies and deeper pressure, negate the need for the incorporation of these techniques into a treatment.

Petrissage – Kneading

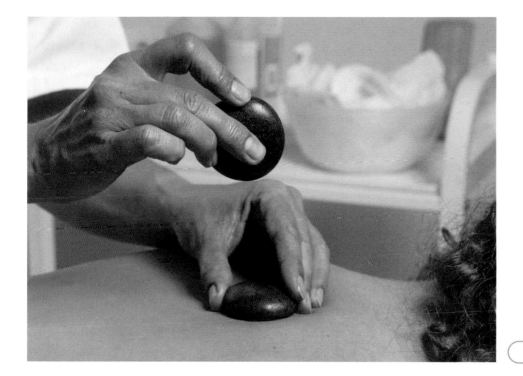

Piezo electric effect

Vibrations
This fine tremulous movement may be performed in several ways.

The side of a stone (hot, cold or one of each) should be held in each hand with the thumbs resting against each other. With the forearms and wrists locked, push the thumbs against each other and the stones down onto the client's skin. Begin a trembling movement from the forearms. The dynamic tension created in the hands should transmit the tremor through to the muscle. Because this is a static movement, ensure that the temperature of the stones is neither too hot, nor cold.

Alternatively, lay the flat side of a stone over the problem area and rhythmically strike it with the side of another: 1,2,3, rest, 1,2,3 rest (or similar) for several sets. The important aspect is that the rhythm remains constant. Excellent for use in relaxation of the muscles; these movements are ideal in preparation for any trigger point work (see below). Use along nerve pathways and/or nerve path endings as this movement will stimulate and clear nerve pathways, due to the 'piezoelectric effect' (see below) in addition to the other effects.

The final way of performing this movement is to rhythmically tap the stones together above one or each chakra, working within the client's aura. The effect of this movement will help balance the chakra and clear the meridians and the aura of negative energies. When working within the aura the temperature of the stones is irrelevant. Only basalt, quartz crystal, or durable stones, measuring six or more on the Moh's scale of hardness should be used for this technique as marble and less dense stones are likely to break.

What is the piezoelectric effect?
The 'piezoelectric effect' is created when the stones are tapped together. The manual pressure on the stones or crystals (ideally quartz) generates a low level electrical current proportional to the stress that they have undergone and a reverberation of penetrative sound waves

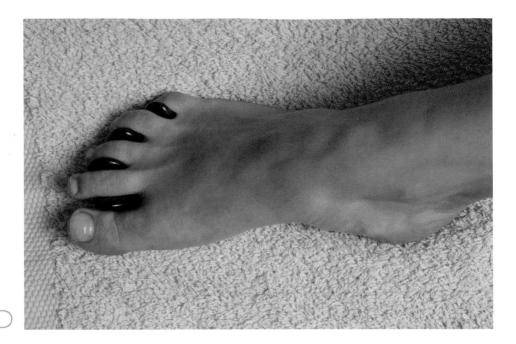

Toe stones

occurs. The result is a powerful and dramatic effect upon the nervous system, bones and muscles.

What is a trigger point?

A trigger point is a hypersensitive, tight, tender, congested part/area of muscle. The problem spot may be full of toxins and waste where there is decreased circulation, increased muscle contraction and/or spasm and nerve sensitivity, ranging from sharp pain to a dull ache. The cause of this may be due to over exercise, trauma, stress or improper warm up prior to exercise.

How can trigger points be helped?

To help ease trigger points use the side or pointed end (in place of the thumb) of a cold stone to apply sustained pressure over the area of inflammation. If the client finds it bearable, this can be done long enough for the muscle to release its spasm. Maintain the pressure until the pain starts to decrease, as this is the trigger point releasing. Slightly increase the pressure as the pain subsides and gradually disperses, then repeat on other areas of muscle and specific adhesions, as necessary. If the area is tense and tight without inflammation, use a hot stone to soothe and warm the area and to relax and lengthen the muscle fibres. If it is too uncomfortable for the client to be worked on directly upon the problem area, then work as closely to it as is possible.

It is important that you gain feedback from the client for this method to work correctly as muscles may be held for anything up to 90 seconds before their trigger point is released.

What are the benefits?

The technique will release the build up of toxins and waste in the muscles helping to restore them to their normal state.

Holding

This is where a stone (usually warm, but not hot) is given to the client to rest in the hands when the client is lying pronate. Other areas to rest the stones would be soles of the feet and backs of the knees as these are all minor chakras and, as such, will help to absorb negative energy.

Pressured Stroking

Use the sides of the stone to 'comb through' the muscle fibres. Use alternate hands to perform this with firm pressure and fairly long, sweeping strokes in the direction of the muscle fibres. This will:

- Increase blood circulation
- Stimulate lymph flow
- Improve muscle tone, with increased elimination of lactic acid build up
- Stimulate the microcirculation to the area
- Stimulate the nervous system

This movement is excellent for lymphatic drainage when performed very lightly, over the surface of the skin. Shorter strokes should be applied in the direction of the nearest lymph node to ensure that lymph does not 'disperse' between strokes. This can help fluid retention and non clinical oedema.

Placement of stones

As part of a treatment, hot and cold stones are often positioned so that the client lies upon them. Various layouts may be adopted depending upon the client's needs and preferences. The important considerations are the effects of using hot and cold stones, so that the appropriate choices are made regarding the outcome of the treatment. Care should be taken to ensure that the stones do not press against bony areas such as the scapula, iliac crest or vertebral column. A towel or cloth should be placed over the stones to prevent burning. Clients find the soothing warmth very relaxing and this can be a very beneficial part of the treatment.

After effects

Often on completion of the treatment, an area may remain reddened. If all guidelines have been followed this will not be the result of a burn, but an indication of congestion in the region or of the muscles concerned or the corresponding organs. This redness will fade over the following twelve to twenty four hours. This after effect should not be used as a diagnostic tool, but a sign that further work may be required.

Where to place the Chakra stones

Basalt stones are high in vibrational energy and, as with crystals, they may be used to balance the chakras. Each of the chakra stones should be placed in turn

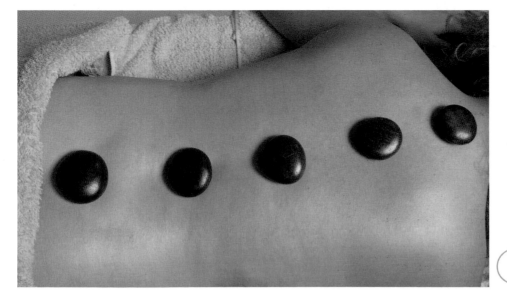

Placement of stones for the spine

STONE THERAPY

onto the body, as the client breathes out (base to crown, to 'wake up'). The removal of the stones should coincide with the client breathing in (crown to base, to 'close down'). Due to the crown chakra being located in the aura, the

stone should be placed to the side of the client on the couch, in line with the top of the head. Likewise, if the third eye stone should fall from its position, place it to the side of the client in line with the third eye chakra.

CARRYING OUT A TREATMENT

What equipment is required?

(See chapter 5 as a guideline for setting up the couch) In addition to this you will need:

- A choice of medium
- A stone heater and thermometer to check the temperature of the stones
- A set of Basalt stones, for heated work – approximately 50 in total. Ideally to include 8 small stones to place between the toes, 7 Chakra stones and a range of large, medium and small stones to use as appropriately for the area concerned.
- Insulated gloves to remove stones from the heater
- Bowl of cold water in which to cool hot stones and occasionally warm frozen stones.
- A set of semi precious gemstones – 7 in total, to include one for each of the chakras as listed previously.
- A set of Marble stones for chilled work: approximately 25 to include a cross section of large, medium and small stones
- A cool box with ice blocks, or some other method of keeping the chilled stones cold
- A receptacle to store used stones until they may be cleaned
- Wooden spoon/spatula for removal of stones

What preparation is required for the client?

The client should be prepared as for massage, having completed a full

consultation, whilst drinking a glass of water (see chapter 5). The client must also be checked for contraindications which are the same as for massage, but with the added consideration of the heat as this will change the dimensions of the treatment. It would therefore be inadvisable to carry out a treatment on clients whose skin:

- Is heat intolerant or hyper sensitive
- Is prone to prickly heat
- Has loss of tactile sensation
- Requires steroid based medication, either orally or topically (skin thinning)
- Has been treated recently with Alpha Hydroxy or Glycolic Acids

In addition to the above, always ensure that the client is not allergic to any of the massage medium ingredients. Obstacles to treatment such as glasses and jewellery should be removed. It is important that an explanation of the treatment be given, including the length of time that it will take, so that the client knows what to expect.

What preparation is required for the therapist?

In addition to the details in chapter 5, the therapist needs to heat the stones to their working temperature of 60 degrees centigrade/140 degrees Fahrenheit. The cold stones should be chilled to 0 degrees centigrade/32 degrees Fahrenheit. It would normally take 30-45 minutes for the stones to reach their desired temperatures. The stones should never be placed in a microwave, or autoclave, as they may explode. Whilst working be aware of posture and ensure that the hands, wrists and joints are kept flexible. The stones should be an extension of the therapist and not held awkwardly. Check the stones for any chips that may scratch the client. When working with energy, it is important that the therapist 'protects' themselves against any negative energies from the client, particularly at the start and closure of a treatment.

Aftercare advice

In addition to normal aftercare (See chapter 5), offer the client a glass of water and allow time for them to 'wake up'. It is not uncommon for the client to feel swings of emotion, as the body readjusts itself and responds to the effects of the treatment. Having stimulated the body systems and 'kick started' the detoxification process it is even more important that the client drinks at least two litres of water a day and avoids drinking tea, coffee and alcohol for the next 24 hours, as the body will be eliminating its toxins and these substances will hinder the process. Light exercise, fresh air and a well balanced diet (to include fresh fruit and vegetables) will help improve general health.

Reactions

Depending upon client reactions, further treatments should be carried out at least one week apart. Common reactions to the treatment include:

- Increased passage of water, defecation, perspiration and mucous production
- Tiredness – the client should respond to how they feel: if tired, rest
- Feeling refreshed and re-energised –

although care should be taken not to do too much
- Healing crisis – the client may feel worse before getting better
- Feelings of euphoria.

Hygiene of the stones

To prevent cross infection all used stones should be cleaned between clients. If any stones have been placed back into the heating unit for reheating during a treatment, then the water should be changed and the heater cleaned with disinfectant too. Alternatively, the use of an oxidiser and sterilising tablet, or solution, in the heating unit will help sanitise the water, until the unit can be thoroughly cleaned and disinfected at the end of the day. Wipe the stones with surgical spirit or alcohol, or antibacterial based solution to remove any medium. Wash in hot soapy water with an antiseptic agent, then rinse until all the soap has gone. This must be carried out after every treatment. If massage medium, particularly oil, is left on marble stones, it will be absorbed. Over a period of time this will soften the stones, causing them to break or chip more easily. In a busy salon or spa setting, ideally two sets of stones should be utilised, so that one kit is being cleaned and prepared, whilst the other is in use. Where crystals have come into contact with the client's skin, they too must be cleaned with hot soapy water and rinsed.

How do we 'cleanse' the stones?

Throughout any treatment the various stones will absorb negative energies. If allowed to build up, the stones will not retain their respective temperatures as efficiently and the treatment will not be so effective. Further negative energies will not be absorbed and the holistic aspect of the treatment will be diminished. The stones must therefore be 'cleansed' or 're-energised'.

Any of the following methods may be adopted for cleansing the crystals and hot and cold stones:

- Expose them to the elements – wind, rain, sun, full moon and thunderstorms; hot stones are recharged better by the sun while crystals and cold stones, by the moon (note that some crystals will fade in sunlight).
- Store them with other crystals such as Labradorite (for either hot or cold) or Moonstone (for cold) until their next use. An amethyst bed is ideal for use with recharging crystals.

- Immerse the stones in sea water, resting them upon natural salt or by sprinkling it over the stones. Never use salt with marble stones or crystals, as it will soften and crack them.
- Use Reiki energy if you are qualified in this therapy
- 'Smudge' the stones with sage incense sticks or store with wild sage
- Using mandalas or medicine wheels (as used by Native Americans)
- Holding the crystals under natural running spring water (specifically) or if this is impractical, soak overnight in bottled mineral water.

You now know what Stone Therapy Massage is, what it does, what the chakras and the aura are, the techniques and equipment required and how to carry out a treatment.

Client Consultation Form – Stone therapy Massage

College Name: Any College
College Number: 123
Student Name: A body
Student Number: 123

Date: Today

Client Name: Mrs Z
Address: Any house, A street
Any Town, Anywhere
Profession: Part time customer care
assisitant

Tel. No: Day 123 456 789
Eve 123 4567

PERSONAL DETAILS

Age group: ☐ Under 20   ☐ 20–30   ☑ 30–40   ☐ 40–50   ☐ 50–60   ☐ 60+
Lifestyle: ☑ Active   ☐ Sedentary
Last visit to the doctor: ☐ 2 months ago
GP Address: The health centre, Get well lane
No. of children (if applicable): 2
Date of last period (if applicable): 3rd day of menstration

CONTRAINDICATIONS REQUIRING MEDICAL PERMISSION – in circumstances where medical permission cannot be obtained clients must give their informed consent in writing prior to treatment (select where/if appropriate):

☐ Pregnancy
☐ Cardiovascular conditions (thrombosis, phlebitis, hypertension, hypotension, heart conditions)
☐ Haemophilia
☐ Any condition already being treated by a GP or another complementary practitioner
☐ Medical oedema
☐ Osteoporosis
☐ Arthritis
☐ Nervous/Psychotic conditions
☐ Epilepsy
☐ Recent operations
☐ Diabetes
☐ Asthma

☐ Any dysfunction of the nervous system (e.g. Multiple sclerosis, Parkinson's disease, Motor neurone disease)
☐ Bell's Palsy
☐ Trapped/Pinched nerve (e.g. sciatica)
☐ Inflamed nerve
☐ Cancer
☐ Postural deformities
☐ Spastic conditions
☐ Kidney infections
☐ Whiplash
☐ Slipped disc
☐ Undiagnosed pain
☐ When taking prescribed medication
☐ Acute rheumatism

CONTRAINDICTIONS THAT RESTRICT TREATMENT (select where/if appropriate):

☐ Fever
☐ Contagious or infectious diseases
☐ Under the influence of recreational drugs or alcohol
☐ Diarrhoea and vomiting
☐ Skin diseases
☐ Undiagnosed lumps and bumps
☐ Localised swelling
☐ Inflammation
☐ Varicose veins
☐ Pregnancy (abdomen)
☐ Cuts
☐ Bruises
☐ Conditions affecting the neck

☐ Abrasions
☐ Scar tissues (2 years for major operation and 6 months for a small scar)
☐ Sunburn
☐ Hormonal implants
☑ Abdomen (first few days of menstruation depending how the client feels)
☐ Haematoma
☐ Hernia
☐ Recent fractures (minimum 3 months)
☐ Cervical spondylitis
☐ Gastric ulcers
☐ After a heavy meal

WRITTEN PERMISSION REQUIRED BY:

☐ GP/Specialist   ☐ Informed consent
Either of which should be attached to the consultation form.

STONE THERAPY

PERSONAL INFORMATION (select if/where appropriate):

Muscular/Skeletal problems: ☑ Back ☑ Aches/Pain ☐ Stiff joints ☑ Headaches
Digestive problems: ☑ Constipation ☑ Bloating ☐ Liver/Gall bladder ☐ Stomach
Circulation: ☐ Heart ☑ Blood pressure ☐ Fluid retention ☑ Tired legs ☑ Varicose veins
☑ Cellulite ☐ Kidney problems ☑ Cold hands and feet
Gynaecological: ☐ Irregular periods ☑ P.M.T ☐ Menopause ☐ H.R.T ☑ Pill ☐ Coil
Nervous system: ☐ Migraine ☑ Tension ☑ Stress ☐ Depression
Immune system: ☐ Prone to infections ☐ Sore throats ☐ Colds ☐ Chest ☑ Sinuses
Regular antibiotic/medication taken? ☐ Yes ☑ No
If yes, which ones: ....
Herbal remedies taken? ☐ Yes ☑ No
If yes, which ones: ....
Ability to relax: ☐ Good ☑ Moderate ☐ Poor
Sleep patterns: ☑ Good ☐ Poor ☐ Average No. of hours 8
Do you see natural daylight in your workplace? ☑ Yes ☐ No
Do you work at a computer? ☑ Yes ☐ No If yes how many hours 3
Do you eat regular meals? ☑ Yes ☐ No
Do you eat in a hurry? ☑ Yes ☐ No
Do you take any food/vitamin supplements? ☑ Yes ☐ No
If yes, which ones: Multi Vitamins ....
How many portions of each of these items does your diet contain per day?
Fresh fruit: 2 Fresh vegetables: 2 Protein: 1 source? Fish or white meat ....
Dairy produce: 4 Sweet things: 2 Added salt: 3 Added sugar: 3
How many units of these drinks do you consume per day?
Tea: 4 Coffee: 4 Fruit juice: 2 Water: 0 Soft drinks: 1 Others: 0
Do you suffer from food allergies? ☐ Yes ☑ No Bingeing? ☐ Yes ☑ No
Overeating? ☐ Yes ☑ No
Do you smoke? ☐ No ☑ Yes How many per day? 1–5
Do you drink alcohol? ☐ No ☑ Yes How many units per day? 2
Do you exercise? ☐ None ☐ Occasional ☑ Irregular ☐ Regular
Types: Aerobics when possible ....
What is your skin type? ☑ Dry ☐ Oil ☐ Combination ☐ Sensitive ☐ Dehydrated
Do you suffer/have you suffered from: ☐ Dermatitis ☐ Acne ☑ Eczema ☐ Psoriasis
☐ Allergies ☑ Hay Fever ☐ Asthma ☐ Skin cancer
Stress level: 1–10 (10 being the highest)
At work 7 At home 5

Reason for treatment: : Mrs Z sometimes experiences 'tension' headaches and often her shoulders and back feel stiff. She would like the treatment to help relieve general aches and pains and allow a little time for relaxation, bringing peace of mind. She has received massage treatments in the past and was curious to experience stone therapy massage to make a comparison between the two for herself. (Throughout the consultation process it was established that the client suffers with congested sinuses, pre menstrual tension, bloating, constipation and cellulite on the upper thigh region. Whilst these problems were not cited as being 'reasons for treatment' upon further discussion my client said that they were areas of concern for her and that she would be happy to receive any treatment that may possibly help to alleviate any or all of these problems.)

REASON FOR TREATMENT

Reason for treatment: Mrs Z sometimes experiences 'tension' headaches and often her shoulders and back feel stiff. She would like the treatment to help relieve general aches and pains and allow a little time for relaxation, bringing peace of mind. She has received massage treatments in the past and was curious to experience stone therapy massage to make a comparison between the two for herself. (Throughout the consultation process it was established that the client suffers with congested sinuses, pre menstrual tension, bloating, constipation and cellulite on the upper thigh region. Whilst these problems were not cited as being 'reasons for treatment' upon further discussion my client said that they were areas of concern for her and that she would be happy to receive any treatment that may possibly help to alleviate any or all of these problems.)

CLIENT PROFILE

Mrs Z is aged 35, a non-smoker, who is happily married with two children aged 7 and 4. She leads a relatively active lifestyle which incorporates walking her children to school and nursery. She enjoys going for family swimming sessions as well as aerobics and tries to attend a class at least once a week. She works part time as a customer care liaison assistant for a large pharmaceutical company, which she finds can be both rewarding and quite frequently, stressful. One evening a week she attends college to study for a qualification linked to her job. Her stress levels for work are higher than she would like, as the nature of her job in itself can be stressful, without the additional pressure of her college course. She attributes her home stress levels to the organisation involved in arranging child care, completing assignments and juggling the various aspects of her everyday life. Her sleep pattern is usually good, although it can be interrupted by the children waking, or occasionally, worry about work. The client is an holistically minded and relatively spiritual person who has received massage treatments in the past. Intermittently she feels that nowadays she has no 'chillout' time and misses this.

She admits that her diet throughout the day could be better, as she often eats food 'on the run', but tries to have a balanced family meal in the evening. At 14 units per week her alcohol intake is just within the ideal guidelines as set for women.

Description of how the therapist conducted the treatment

Having completed the consultation it was established that Mrs Z had no contraindications requiring medical permission, or restrictions that would affect the treatment. Once helped and settled onto the couch, I ensured that the client was both supported and comfortable. I sanitised the client's feet and washed my hands. Tactile and thermal sensitivity tests were then conducted upon all areas to be massaged. It was concluded that Mrs Z's reactions were normal which meant that a full stone therapy treatment could go ahead.

The lighting was dimmed, with the room being both quiet and warm. Gentle music was played in the background. The treatment was explained to the client with time allowed for her to ask questions. The basalt stones and their heater had been cleaned and positioned

STONE THERAPY

in readiness for the treatment (temperature at approximately 140 degrees fahrenheit) whilst the cold marble stones had been sprayed with sterilising solution and lay on a bed of ice (temperature approximately 32 degrees fahrenheit).

A visualisation technique was used to help her to relax, yet focus upon the treatment. During this process I prepared and protected myself against any potentially negative energies released from the client. I commenced the treatment with the client lying prone, by performing several techniques designed to 'wake up' the chakras and placed the following semi precious gem stones, beneath the couch, in line with their respective chakras: root chakra - garnet, sacral chakra - carnelian, solar plexus - tiger's eye, heart chakra - green tourmaline, throat chakra - lapis lazuli, 3rd eye chakra - fluorite and crown chakra - amethyst.

Warm foot covers were laid over the client's feet and I wrapped the largest of the hot basalt stones in one layer of towelling and placed this over the client's sacral region. This would diffuse warmth throughout the area and help to release any tension, preparing the area for deeper massage.

I proceeded to carry out the full massage routine making the following amendments and changes:

Whilst working on Mrs Z's back, tension was felt in the erector spinae muscle between the scapulae, with nodules and adhesions being apparent in the trapezius muscle and tension up into splenius capitis. To address this problem more kneading and wringing movements were carried out with hot stones. Frictions and cross fibre frictions were then performed on the problem areas (using marble stones) before returning to the heated stones once again. The piezoelectric technique was applied on the erector

spinae (being mindful to protect and not work upon the vertebral column) using basalt stones followed by deep stroking, to help disperse the tension. This rhythmical tapping technique was also utilised on the tension nodules of the trapezius, but with more force, before using a deep stroking movement with one warm stone to work along the fibres of the muscle. An extra set of vibrations was carried out either side of the vertebral column to stimulate and have a knock-on relaxation effect to the nerves. The piezoelectric effect was also incorporated over the same area. The massage ended with effleurage of the whole back. The client was then asked to turn over and helped to a sitting position with her modesty intact.

A glass of water was provided for Mrs Z to drink whilst the stones were strategically positioned on the bed for her to lie upon. Six pairs of hot stones were positioned within the thoracic region (being mindful of the vertebral column) with the top two pairs of stones being marble. A cloth was laid over the stones and the client helped to gently lay down. After checking Mrs Z's comfort, the toe stones were placed between her toes, with a small basalt stone being held in each of her hands. Two small stones were placed behind each knee. One large basalt stone was placed on each of the first five chakras as the client breathed out, with a cold marble stone being placed on the 3rd eye chakra and at the head of the bed for the crown chakra. No alteration was made to the normal routine whilst working on the arms and hands, except that I forgot to perform the 'closing down' chakra sequence on both hands. This was remedied later when I performed the closing sequence on the feet.

Massage of the abdominal region was omitted due to the client having commenced menstruation. The time that would have been spent on this region was devoted to reworking the problem areas, as described.

The toe stones were removed from between the toes and there were no adaptations to the massage routine for the feet. Pressure circles were used on the chakra points of the foot to close them down (then on the hands) and the closing techniques for the whole treatment were performed. This included the incorporation of the piezoelectric/tapping effect using each of the chakra stones (one upon the other within the auric field) from crown to base. The routine was now complete and any remaining stones were removed. On inspection of the client's back, four areas of erythema were apparent where the client had lain on the heated stones. (This may indicate areas of congestion and tension, which would benefit from further work.) Interestingly, there were no areas of redness where the lowest pair of heated stones had been, or the cool marble stones. The client was given a glass of water to drink whilst discussing the aftercare advice.

Rationale for choice of treatment

A stone massage treatment will provide a deeper pressure and penetration of heat to soothe muscular aches and pains. It also allows for maximum relaxation and balance on a physical, psychological and spiritual level.

The massage medium chosen was jojoba. This is a light, nutritive, water soluble oil, resembling sebum and mimicking collagen.It remains stable under heat thereby allowing the stones to move easily over an area without becoming sticky and will benefit Mrs Z's dry skin. The heat from the stones will allow for deeper absorption of the oil, helping to moisturise the skin.

Due to my client being spiritually minded, the use of gem stones and various techniques to open, balance and close the chakras, as well as clear the auric field were discussed and utilised. It was decided to incorporate these procedures as they may help to uplift and clear Mrs Z's mind, enabling her to focus on any tasks ahead. She may possibly feel more emotionally balanced and re-energised. The respective gem stones were chosen in association with their corresponding chakra to help balance them, by strengthening weaker areas and neutralising dominant ones.

When performing effleurage, wringing and kneading movements the stones were held flat in the palms of the hands, allowing for deeper pressure.

The sides of the stones or 'lighthouse' shaped stones were used for frictions, cross fibre frictions, trigger points work and drainage movements. Again, this provides a deeper more concentrated pressure, whilst protecting the therapist's thumbs, wrist joints and fingers.

The piezoelectric effect was incorporated directly onto the body to resonate through the internal organs and help release the stubborn trigger points in the trapezius and levator scapula muscles. When utilised in the aura, hovering over each of the chakras, it has a dramatic effect on the nervous and endocrine systems. It is thought that this will help 'clear' the auric field and rebalance the chakras.

Small heated stones were given to the client to hold in the palm of her hand and placed behind the knee in the popliteal region, as these are secondary chakras and may help to absorb any negative energies. Basalt stones were placed on each of the first 5 chakras in turn, so that the vibrational energy of the hot stones would resonate with the energy of the chakras and help balance them. This may help the client to feel more calm and emotionally balanced.

How the client felt during the treatment

The client said that throughout the treatment she felt warm and contented. She seemed happy with the pressure and said "ooh that feels good" as I worked over the areas of tension on her back. Initially, she was slightly apprehensive of lying on the back placement stones, as she thought that they would be uncomfortable, but was surprised at how relaxing it was. Soon afterwards she said that she could not tell that cold stones had been included at all.

How the client felt after the treatment

Mrs Z reported that she felt totally relaxed and less stressed. Her mind felt "chilled out, but clear" and she felt safe to drive home. Her shoulders and neck she thought were much "looser than before, with easier mobility". She said that she had really enjoyed the treatment and that it felt quite different to normal massage, as well as to how she imagined it would be, having seen pictures of stone placements in various magazines. The piezoelectric effect she said had felt "strange and unusual, but not in a bad way, just different...." She also said that she enjoyed the depth of the massage combined with the heat and that she was already looking forward to the next treatment.

Home care advice given

The date for a follow on treatment was discussed and it was decided that to gain maximum benefit, the client should attend a further treatment in one week's time and continue with weekly treatments for the next 3 sessions then reassess the situation. Ideally, as time progresses and the client's problems improve, it was explained that a monthly maintenance treatment would be a model scenario, with extra visits as and when the client felt it necessary. The treatment can have a very powerful effect on the emotions and I advised the client that in the short term she and/or her husband may notice a change in mood, but that this would even out over the next 24-48 hours. Additionally, the body may try to eliminate waste, so this was outlined to the client. Occasionally, it was explained that clients may feel worse before they feel better, again this reaction is not uncommon, but will happen less and less with each treatment. When working on the computer at work and/or at home I suggested that she try to take small breaks, or at least stretch out her shoulders and arms (which I demonstrated to her).

Reflective practice

On reflection I feel that the treatment went very well. I remembered my routine except for the closing down chakra movements on both hands and was able to use my knowledge to adapt it to the client's needs. I feel that I explained the treatment well to Mrs Z, especially as she had shown such interest in the chakras and aura. She wanted to know how and why the techniques used could influence these areas (body, mind and spirit). Having treated this client previously, I was aware of how open to the concept of clearing the auric field and balancing the chakras she would be. However, with other clients I am very conscious of their potential scepticism and must remember that not all people would subscribe to these theories. I need to gauge whether a client would be comfortable with this or whether it would be better to provide a stone massage treatment, which would produce benefits from the use of the stones and alternating temperatures alone. I must always ensure that if I open and balance the chakras for a client they must be closed properly as well to prevent the client from feeling 'spaced out'. I feel that I should have given the client more aftercare advice, but did not want to bombard her with information and I think that I covered the most important points. However, I must remember to mention the additional things at our next meeting.

Overall conclusion of case study

I think that this treatment was ideal for Mrs Z in that she needed some rest and relaxation time. She appeared to be far less stressed having received the treatment and definitely lucid. It would appear that the tension in her back and shoulders has been alleviated to a certain extent. It could be said that Mrs Z appeared to be a 'fan' of stone therapy massage, so the main objectives of the treatment had been achieved.

TREATMENT 2

Description of how the therapist conducted the treatment

I checked to ensure that Mrs Z's medical details had not changed from the previous week's consultation. She confirmed that the only change was that she had now finished menstruating and would like to experience the abdominal massage this week. She also reported that after last weeks treatment she had felt revitalised, being able to whizz through the housework and chores with more vigour, but subsequently felt extremely tired by the end of the day. She said that her back neck and shoulders felt so much better, even after she had been to work the next day, but the aches and pains had since returned. She said that she had experienced a few of the 'elimination' side effects mentioned previously and was glad that she had been made aware of them. Currently she had been feeling a little discomfort from abdominal bloating. Her stress levels had slightly improved from the previous week, but there was no particular reason for this. She had not experienced any headaches this week which she was pleased about.

Due to the apparent success of the first treatment, it was decided that a similar treatment be repeated and all aspects were carried out as before with the following amendments:

I reworked all of the areas, as described in the first routine, but for less time as massage of the abdomen was to be included.

The tension in my clients upper back had improved and the knots were not so apparent, so the additional movements were carried out as previously described, but with fewer repetitions, again reducing time. However, this week there appeared to be more tension in the lumbar region and gluteus medius, so extra petrissage movements of wringing, kneading and frictions were carried out, to help ease this tension. When the time came for the spinal layout I chose to use all heated stones and placed four more pairs further down her back, instead of incorporating the cold stones. However, this time I placed cold stones for Mrs Z to hold in her hands for the duration of the massage of the head and neck, before changing them to warm.

The scalp did not seem so tight this week, and the skin moved more freely as I worked. Less circling (shampooing) repetitions were carried out. The marble stone that I placed on the 3rd eye chakra kept falling off, so I exchanged it for a warm stone instead and it remained in place. When carrying out the facial drainage movements, the pressure used was light. I alternated the use of warm and cold stones.

Pressure was greatly reduced also whilst working over the abdominal region. Having previously warmed the area with the use of hot stones for effleurage and petrissage movements, a cold stone was used for kneading the abdomen following the direction of the colon. This was repeated with a heated stone, then alternate stroking using both a hot and cold stone over the acending transverse and descending colon. I was careful to watch my client's reactions, to ensure that there was no discomfort, but she said that the pressure was fine. I rested four small cold stones in isolation along the transverse colon region whilst preparing the legs for massage, then removed them, lightly stroking the area briefly with a heated stone before performing final effleurage movements. From this point on the treatment followed the usual routine with no further additionalities.

Rationale for choice of treatment

The client's needs were very similar to the first treatment, except that she also had some lower back ache this week and abdominal massage was to be included. The theory for the use of the stones was followed, but heated stones were used for the spinal layout without the incorporation of the cold for this treatment, as there appeared to be less inflammation in the trapezius and levator scapula muscles and more tension in quadratus lumborum. The heated stone placements were continued further down her back than before, to have an effect upon the lower areas of tension. It would be inadvisable to use cold stones for a long duration in this lower back area (i.e. with the client lying upon them) due to the position of the kidneys, but the use of the heated stones would help to disperse the tension

without potentially creating problems. The frictions and cross fibre frictions on the lower back muscles were carried out, alternating the use of cold and heated stones to increase circulation.

Initially, having turned Mrs Z over, I gave her a cold stone to hold in each hand, as a short application (held marble stones) may help to affect the organs of the body, increasing contraction of the muscles in the abdominal region. This was with a view to easing the bloated feeling and helping her body find it's natural rhythm again. A heated stone then replaced the cold for client comfort. Although, the client had not had any headaches this week, I was still going to incorporate a cool stone on her 3rd eye chakra, as it feels soothing. It would appear however that it was not required, as it kept falling off. The use of the warmed basalt stone would help to balance the chakra instead. Throughout the facial massage pressure was light, so that the skin was not dragged in any way. I alternated the use of warm and cold stones on the face to help stimulate the area and remove any toxins, but changed them for cold at my client's request. A short application of cold stones directly over the large intestine area will help to increase peristaltic movement whilst massage using a cold stone will stimulate and aid peristalsis. This will hopefully help to improve Mrs Z's constipation.

How the client felt during the treatment

Mrs Z appeared to relax very quickly into the treatment and she almost seemed to drift off to sleep, as I worked on her back. She appeared to particularly enjoy the extra work carried out over the lower back region, as she commented that she had been "overdoing the gardening and was now paying the price." She also said that she enjoyed the abdominal massage more than she expected and that none of the movements made her feel uncomfortable. This was a concern of mine as her tummy appeared to be a little swollen today and Mrs Z had confirmed that she was feeling slightly bloated.

How the client felt after the treatment

Mrs Z said that she had really enjoyed the treatment and felt very calm "light in her body and mind", but invigorated. She felt that she had been able to forget the problems she had been thinking about more and more as the treatment progressed. The aches in her back seemed to be much improved and she had decided that she liked "the tapping thing" (piezoelectric effect). She also said that she felt quite thirsty, which prompted me to fetch her a glass of water and we discussed the after care advice. Mrs Z said that whilst she still enjoyed massage, she felt that the incorporation of the stones definitely enhanced the treatment making it much more effective.

Have care advice given

The homecare provided for last week's treatment was reiterated, but I stressed that even if Mrs Z should feel invigorated and full of energy, it would be wise not to do too much and have a more relaxing day following this treatment, than cleaning the house. To help with her shoulder tension I suggested that she check whether the height and/or position of her desk and computer were comfortable, or whether this could be contributing to her problems. Mrs Z sometimes works for fairly long durations at the computer and confirmed that it did not have an anti-glare visa in place. I therefore suggested that she check with work to see whether one could be fitted, as this may affect her headaches, or alternatively, I suggested

that she try wearing sunglasses whilst on the computer, to see if this made any difference. In addition to drinking more water, I suggested that she have a glass of prune juice in the morning to help with the constipation. An appointment was arranged for her next visit in a week's time as agreed previously.

Reflective practice

Again, I feel that this treatment went well. I remembered to close down the chakras in each of the relevant places of the routine this time. It was gratifying to know that Mrs Z had listened to and acted upon my previous aftercare advice, so that I felt confident in providing her with further information. In future when placing stones on a particular region i.e. 3rd eye, I will not waste time trying to keep the stone in place if it keeps falling off, as this breaks the continuity of the treatment. I will change it once for a stone of the opposite temperature, but if this does not work I will simply place it to the side of the area, in line with the respective chakra and continue with the treatment. Treating this client has helped me to consolidate my routine, so that I am now more flowing in the movements.

Overall conclusion of case study

This stone therapy massage has been appropriate to Mrs Z's needs and the results have been very encouraging. Her muscular aches and pains have been relieved somewhat and the areas of tension seem less tight. She enjoyed the abdominal massage which may also help her constipation, so the client's needs have been met. Psychologically, there appears to have been an improvement in Mrs Z's outlook that sceptics could attribute to having taken the time to relax and unwind, however I feel that the 'holistic' nature of this treatment has given my client a boost in body, mind and spirit.

TREATMENT 3

Description of how the therapist conducted the treatment:

I checked to ensure that Mrs Z's medical details had not changed from the previous week's consultation. She confirmed that this was the case, but she had experienced a few headaches this week which she attributed to stress at work. After last week's treatment she was happy to report that her abdominal bloating had been alleviated. She was concerned however, about the areas of cellulite on her thighs and wondered whether special consideration could be given to this. I therefore chose a professional range anti cellulite cream as the medium for the upper leg massage (front and back) and jojoba for the rest of the body.

I proceeded to carry out the full massage routine making the following amendments and changes:

Mrs Z had relatively toned leg muscles and I was able to apply deeper effleurage movements, than with previous clients. Once the area had been warmed, I performed extra petrissage movements with the stones. Kneading and wringing techniques using heated stones were carried out, paying particular attention to the areas of cellulite. I then held one hot and one cold stone in each hand and used these alternately (with each stroke) to work along the fibres of the hamstring muscles. There appeared to be tension both here and in the calf muscles, so extra friction and cross fibre frictions were incorporated to disperse the tension (initially using a marble stone, then a basalt stone). A warm stone was held and used with firm pressure to travel the length of the muscle from start to finish, again to help disperse the tension. The stones were used in small circular motions over the cellulite with a firm, but comfortable pressure (initially cold, then hot). Light drainage movements, using

alternate cold and hot stones were stroked toward the inguinal nodes, as this would be beneficial for the cellulite and removal of toxins. I finalised the movements for this area with effleurage and removed the foot warmers.

Similar movements were carried out upon the lower leg, with small stones being used to lightly massage the sides of the achilles tendon. Any drainage movements were directed towards the popliteal lymph nodes behind the knee.

When I commenced working on the scalp and throughout this part of the treatment I carried out extra circling (shampooing) movements with hot stones as the skin felt tight. Whilst completing the face and front of neck massage I incorporated more lymph drainage movements over the sinuses and down to the clavicles with the sides of two marble stones working simultaneously, as opposed to alternating the stones with warm.

Whilst working over the chest and shoulders heated stones were used on their sides to stroke up and down the muscle fibres of trapezius. A firm pressure was used on the posterior compartment, but this was drastically reduced when combing through the muscle fibres of the anterior compartment. This was repeated with a cold stone, then once more with a heated one.

The increased movements performed on the backs of the legs were adopted for the front of the legs with the additon of circular movements of small heated stones around the patella and drainage to the back of the knee.

Throughout all three treatments I checked with my client that the pressure was neither too light nor too heavy and that the stones used were neither too hot nor too cold. Every time I removed a stone from the heater I was careful to ensure that the reading on the thermometer was approximately 140 degrees fahrenheit, but no higher. If the stones felt a little warm I would turn them in my hands, to absorb some of the heat before applying them to the skin. When stones were too hot I quickly dipped them in and out of a bowl of cold water, until they felt at a comfortable temperature.

Rationale for choice of treatment:

The anti-cellulite cream was chosen as a medium because it remains stable under heat and is beneficial for this area. The choice and use of the stones is as follows: One stroke with a heated basalt stone is thought to be the equivalent of 10 manual massage strokes. The metabolism of an area is stimulated, increasing the local body temperature and promoting the rate of tissue repair. By incorporating heated stones, benefits to the client are achieved more quickly with tired aching muscles being returned to their normal state more readily. The warmth from the stones, softens the tissues, so that deeper more penetrative work can be achieved more rapidly, bringing faster relief with less work on the part of the therapist.

The utilisation of cold marble stones into the treatment will reduce the microcirculation, cooling, soothing and desensitising the area to help reduce pain, hence the use of a cold stone on the 3rd eye chakra to help with headaches. The flesh will be tightened and firmed when using cold stones and the decongestant action means that they were ideal for use on the client's face. The stones were used to help drain blocked sinuses by helping to decongest blocked passages. Cold marble stones will reduce inflammation, which is why they were used on the tension areas and trigger points of the trapezius and levator scapula. The tension build up in this area, could well be the cause of Mrs Z's aches and pains in the upper back, neck and shoulders as well as contributing to her tension headaches. Application of cold massage stones were used for approximately half the time of the heated, as they may have begun to feel uncomfortable or could even have caused a burn.

The use of alternate hot and cold stones in an area will help to increase circulation and lymph flow in a 'stop start fashion' to 'flush out' toxins. This is why this technique was employed for the client's cellulite and for trigger points work. However, the final strokes were always carried out using a heated stone, for client comfort and to return the skin back to its normal temperature.

How the client felt during the treatment

Mrs Z appeared very relaxed. She thought that the use of the cool stones seemed refreshing and stimulating rather than the shock to the system she thought it would initially be. Again she almost seemed to drift off to sleep. She particularly enjoyed the head, face and neck movements saying that it was almost as if the tension was "draining away". Mrs Z thought that the movements and pressure over her areas of cellulite were good and hoped that it would make a difference! She felt that the movements either side of her ankle (Achilles tendon movement) felt "very nice and soothing".

How the client felt after the treatment

Mrs Z said that the use of the chilled stones on her face felt quite exhilarating and was something she had not experienced before. She commented that she preferred the feeling of cool stones in the facial massage, as opposed to warm, or alternating warm and cool. She requested a tissue (as the decongestant action of the cold stones in the facial routine had already started the elimination process) .She had really enjoyed the treatment and said that her legs "felt light." She felt that she had been able to forget her problems and that her head seemed clear. I fetched a glass of water and we discussed her after care advice.

Homecare advice given

The homecare provided for the previous week's treatments were reiterated. I was quick to explain that no change in the appearance of her cellulite would be apparent yet and that she would need to attend regular treatments to make any difference. Other things that she may consider that would also have a positive effect, would be cutting down on the amount of tea, coffee and alcohol drunk. (In fact all of these should be avoided for at least the next 24 hours to obtain maximum benefit from the treatment.) I asked her to try to drink more water to help the elimination process (at least 2 litres per day) using diluted cordial if that would help the taste. I advised that it would be very common for the body to try and expel anything it didn't need, so it would be normal to go to the toilet more, perspire, cough or expel phlegm along with any other ways that the body may rid itself of waste. A demonstration of 'dry skin brushing ' was given and I suggested that Mrs Z perform this morning and night, if possible, after having massaged the cellulitic area (the more, the better). I proposed that she try to cut down on the amount of refined, processed food, salt and sugar consumed and eat more natural foodstuffs such as fruit and vegetables. I spoke to her about galvanic treatments which would also help in the treatment of cellulite and details of how this would work. (A referral was made to a body therapist to discuss the benefits and possible appointment times.)

Alternatively, I suggested that she try wearing sun glasses whilst on the computer, to see if this made any difference.

Reflective practice

Again, I feel that this treatment went well. I remembered to close down the chakras in each of the relevant places in the routine this time.I must always ensure that if I open and balance the chakras for a client they must be closed properly as well to prevent the client from feeling 'spaced out'. I enjoyed carrying out this treatment, as my client's needs gave me the chance to try out the varying techniques in full, whereas previously on clients I had practised massaging the body using the stones in a relatively traditional way, rather than 'holistically'. There is something satisfying about carrying out the piezoelectric effect and I really enjoy performing it. I feel that I am now becoming more familiar with the way the stones sit in my hands when perfoming effleurage, so that I no longer hold the stones, but push them as if they were an extension of my own hand. It was gratifying to know that Mrs Z had listened to and acted upon my previous aftercare advice, so that I felt confident in providing her with further information. I think that because she enjoys swimmimg and is obviously conscious of her cellulite, she seemed genuinely pleased to be referred to a colleague who would be able to help carry out further different work on the area. Treating this client has helped me to consolidate my routine and given me ample opportunity to hone my skills as a stone massage therapist, with techniques such as frictions, cross fibre frictions and piezoelectric movements.

Overall conclusion of case study

I think that this course of treatments were ideal for Mrs Z in that her main objectives have been addressed. She needed some rest and relaxation time whilst alleviating the knots and adhesions, evident in her tired muscles. The fact that Mrs Z wanted to blow her nose at the end of this treatment was a positive sign that her congested sinuses were clearing. Her body was already responding to and becoming more proficient at eliminating waste, which will be of all round benefit. She is more positive in her outlook, with the treatments having lessened her general aches, pains and tension and reduced her headaches. Having enjoyed being a case study she is keen to continue with stone massage as well as being referred for additonal treatments in relation to her cellulite. I feel that with following the aftercare advice and continuing with ongoing treatment plans, a marked improvement in her cellulite will be seen, as well as in providing the deep sense of relaxation and psychological 'lift' that the client has experienced with geothermotherapy - stone therapy massage.

HOT STONES MASSAGE ROUTINE

Stones needed for the Massage Routine

1 x Large Sacral Chakra Stone
4 x Stones for working on the side of the body (Bag 1)
4 x Stone for working on the back of the legs (Bag 2)
4x   Slightly larger stones for working on the back (Bag 3)
8 x Stones for lying under the clients back (Bag 4)
7 x Chakra stones, 5 large and 2 small to lay on the client's body (Bag 5)
8 x Cosy Ice Stones (Green Net)
6 x Small stones, 2 stones to place in the hands, 2 stones to place behind the knees and 2 face stones (Bag 6)
4 x Chest Stones
4 x Stones for the legs (Bag 8)

Overview of the sequence of the areas of the body to work on

1) Lay the client on their front
2) Place the Chakra crystals in place on the floor under the treatment couch.
3) Place the Sacral Chakra stone in place
4) Rock the back
5) Commence the treatment at the Crown Chakra
6) Work on the right side of the body, then the left side of the body
7) Work on the back of the legs
8) Work on the back
9) Turn the client over
10) Sit the client up and place the 8 stones in place for the back
11) Place the Chakra stones on the front of the client's body beginning with the Root Chakra Stone.
12) Place the cosy toes stones in place.
13) Place hot stones into the palm of each hand and behind each knee.
14) Work on the scalp
15) Work on the face
16) Work on the chest, shoulders and the back of the neck
17) Work on the hands and arms
18) Work on the front of the legs
19) Work on the feet
20) Close the Chakras down with the removal of the stones
21) Remove any stones on or around the client
22) Remove the crystals placed on the floor.

Have a bowl of cool water to one side in case any of the stones need cooling before they are used.

STONE THERAPY

WORKING ON THE BACK OF THE BODY

Stones needed when working on the back of the body.

- *Large Sacral Chakra Stone*
- *4 stones for working on the sides of the body. (Bag 1)*
- *4 Stones for working on the legs. (Bag 2)*
- *4 slightly larger stones for working on the back. (bag 3)*
- *2 cloths.*

1) Begin by positioning the client face up on the couch if you need to remove any make-up from the client's face. Then ask the client to turn over so they are lying on their front.
(if there is not a face hole in the couch, give the client a support for their head.)

2) Begin by positioning the client face up on the couch. Then ask the client to turn over so they are lying on their front.
(if there is not a face hole in the couch, give the client a support for their head.)
3) Take the Sacral Chakra stone out of the heater and wrap it in a small hand towel. Place the stone at the base of the client's back in line with their sacrum.
4) Unwrap the 4 stones to start the routine (bag 1) and place them inside the warm towel.
5) Wring out the foot protectors and shake the excess heat out of them. Check the temperature is suitable for the client then place them over the client's feet.
6) Place the crystals on the ground under the client's body in line with their 7 major Chakras.

CROWN CHAKRA

7) Go to the head of the bed and prepare yourself and the client for the routine.
8) Stand with your feet shoulder width apart
9) Close your eyes and concentrate on your breathing
10) Rub your hands together and try and concentrate on nothing other than a bright white light and your own steady breathing
11) Stop rubbing your hands together and open your eyes, gently move your hands towards the clients Crown Chakra
12) Holding your hands either in the clients aura or making contact with the physical body, ask the client to concentrate on their breathing, try to balance your breathing with your client's breathing.

13) Ask your client to try to imagine a bright white light comes and to keep returning to this when other come into their mind.

Stand on the side of the client and place one hand on the Chakra stone and the other between the client's shoulder blades. Gently rock the client horizontally for a few seconds while concentrating on your breathing. Now place one hand on one of your client's shoulders and your other hand on the client's opposite hip, rock horizontally for a few seconds and then repeat on the other side.

Remove the heated foot covers from the client's feet and dry them.

RIGHT SIDE OF THE BODY

14) Uncover the right side of the client's body exposing their right leg, right arm and right side of their back. Take 2 medium sized stones and place them on the couch at the sides of the client's leg. Warm your hands on the stones and then apply a small amount of oil to the right side of the body.

15) Start at the ankle, move up to the knee, when on the back of the knee turn your body and the stones so that you are pulling the stones up the client's hamstrings to the top of the leg.

16) Slide the stones over to the palm of the client's hand, keep one of your hands on the stone in the client's hand and move the other stone in your other hand up the arm and top of the shoulder.

17) Gently slide down the back and down the back and down the leg returning to the ankle.

Repeat twice then turn the stones over and repeat twice.

LEFT SIDE OF THE BODY

18) Cover the right side of the body and then uncover the left side of the body exposing their left leg, left arm and left side of the back. Take 2 medium sized stones and place them on the couch at the sides on the client's leg. Warm your hands on the stones and then apply a small amount of oil to the right side of the body.

- Start at the ankle, move up to the knee, when on the back of the knee turn your body and the stones so that you are pulling the stone's up the client's hamstrings to the top of the leg.

- Slide the stones over to the palm of the client's hand, keep one of your hands on the stone in the client's hand and move the other stone in your other hand up the arm and on to the top of the shoulder.

- Gently slide down the back and down the leg returning to the ankle.

- Repeat twice then turn the stones over and repeat twice again.

19) Cover the left side of the body then remove 4 stones for the legs (bag 2)

and place them inside the warm towel.

20) Uncover the bottom of both legs to the level of the knees. Place 2 of the hot stones at the back of the clients knees on top of the towel. Effleurage both the calves simultaneously including the Achilles tendon and the sides of the heels. Turn the stones over and Petrissage (pressure circles) either side of the calf and then up the centre of the calf.

21) Uncover the top of both legs to the level of the buttocks. Take 2 hot stones and place one on each buttock, on top of the towel. Effleurage oil over the hamstring, then up the middle. Effleurage the full leg once then leave the hot stones on the client's feet.

22) Cover the client's legs then take the 4 back stones out of the water heater (Bag 3) and wrap them in the towel ready for use.

23) Move the Sacral Chakra stone and place it at the base of the bottom, between the legs.

BACK

24) Uncover the client's back and place 2 of the stones at the side of the client's shoulders. Standing at the head of the bed warm your hands with the heat of the stones and apply a small amount of the massage oil over the client's back and arms. Using 2 stones effleurage down the spine up the sides of the body and then down the upper arm to the level of the elbow then break contact with the client.

Move to the base of the back and turn the stones over, work up the sides of the spine, across the upper fibres of Trapezius and then down the arms and off the palms x 4.

Change the stones for 2 more hot ones and standing at the side of the bed effleurage the trapezius and round the scapula. Petrissage the area right around the scapula (for the clients with problems in this area you can out their arms into the small of their back to open up the Scapula). Friction movements can be used on areas of muscle tensions and adhesions.

Turn the stones over and work over the area of the sacrum and out over the gluteals firstly with effleurage and then Petrissage.

Use vibration movements up or down each side of the spine (up for uplifting – down to calm down)

Finish the back with sweeping movements again either up or down each side of the spine using the sides of the stones x 3.

25) Cover the clients back and remove any remaining stones.
(Unwrap the stone that was covering the Sacral Chakra and put it back in the water heater).

TURN THE CLIENT OVER

Stones needed when working on the front of the body:

- *8 Stones to lie under the client's back (Bag 4)*
- *7 Chakra stones, 5 large and 2 small (Bag 5)*
- *8 Cosy toe Stones (Green Net)*
- *2 stones to place in the hands, 2 stones to place behind the knees and 2 face stones (Bag 6)*
- *4 Chest Stones (Bag 7)*
- *4 Stones for the legs (Bag 8)*
- *1 Cloth*

Remove the following stones from the water heater:
- *Stones for the back (Bag 4)*
- *Chakra Stones (Bag 5)*

- *Cosy Toes*
- *Stones for placing in the client's hands (Bag 6)*
- *Stones for placing behind the client's knees (Bag 6)*
- *Stones for the face (Bag 6)*
- *Wrap them in the towel ready for use.*

Carefully sit the client up leaving the bed flat. Place the 8 stones on the bed so that they will be positioned either side of the spine on the Erector Spinae Muscles, work from the bottom of the back up to the level of the Scapula. Cover the stones with a towel then gently lay the client back on the stones. Ensure the client is comfortable, the stones should not be too hot or catching the bones of the spine.

Place the 7 Chakra stones on the front of the client, beginning with the root chakra down at the base of the pelvis or just below (do not place the stones directly onto the genitalia). Place all of the remaining stones on the Chakras ensuring the smaller stone for the Third Eye Chakra is placed on top of the cloth. Place the stone for the Crown Chakra just above the client's head on the bed. (Co-ordinate the placing of the stones with the client exhaling).

PUT IN THE COSY TOES STONES

26) Take the 8 cosy toes stones (Green net) and beginning by the little toe, place them in between each of the toes.
27) Take the stones from the Bag 6 and place one into the palm of each hand and one behind each knee (check these stones are not too hot: cool them in water if they are).

Scalp

28) Position yourself at the head of the bed: you may prefer to sit for this part of the treatment (you can elevate the head of the bed or put a pillow under the client's head if they do not like to be completely flat).

Remove the stone and the cloth from the Third eye Chakra.

Take 2 small stones (the one placed at the Crown Chakra and the one at the Third eye Chakra) and place them into the palms of your hands. Begin to circle the stones on the head gently (like a shampooing movement). First turn the head to one side so you can work behind it, then turn the head to the other side to get right behind it. After a minute turn the stones over. Make sure the whole of the head is covered. Put the stones to the side of the head and comb your fingers up through the hair, working right to the tips of the hair.

Face and front of the neck.

29) Take 2 smaller stones (bag 6) and ensuring that they are not too hot begin at the centre of the forehead. Apply pressure point work from the centre of the eyebrows up the forehead and back over the head to the crown. Then perform draining movements out from the centre of the face to the outside, always moving towards a lymph node. (Cover the whole face) Continue this movement right down the sides of the neck to the clavicles and complete with drainage movements from the corners of the mandible down the sides of the neck to the clavicles.

Remove 4 stones (bag 7) from the heater and wrap them in the towel to keep them warm. Place the stone from the Throat Chakra to one side of throat on the bed and lower the towel.

CHEST AND SHOULDERS/ARMS AND HANDS

3) Take 2 stones (Bag 7) and effleurage across the chest, down the arms to the elbows and back up and over the deltoids. Once on the point of the shoulders stand the stones on their sides and draw them in over the trapezius and up the sides of the neck, repeat x 6.

Take 2 new stones (Bag 7); place them under the upper fibres of the trapezius. Turn the head to one side, take the stone from under the side of the trapezius that is exposed and work with the side of the stone from the shoulder in and up the neck and back again. Keep rotating the stones to work with warm edges. Place the stone back under the trapezius when you have completed the work on that side.

Arms and Hands

31) Move to the client's right hand and hold it firmly with one hand and knead the stone the client was holding into the palm of the hand. Using the side of the stone effleurage from the wrist down the forearm to the inside of the elbow x 4 then repeat on the posterior surface of the forearm. Put the stones down firmly wring the hand then working with your thumb work from the Crown Chakra down the side of the thumb to the Root Chakra to close the Chakras down

Repeat the procedure on the left hand.

FRONT OF LEGS/FEET

Remove 4 stones (bag 8) from the heater and wrap them in the towel, ready for use.

32) Uncover the lower half of the client's legs, up to the level of the knees. Place 2 of the hot stones between the client's legs on top of the towel. Effleurage the lower part of both legs simultaneously and the sides of the ankles. Petrissage (pressure circles) either side of the tibia.

33) Uncover the top of both legs to the level of the groin. Take 2 hot stones and place them on the lower abdomen, on top of the towel. Effleurage over the thighs then turn the stones over and Petrissage up the outside, then up the inside (use less pressure here) and then up the middle of the thighs. Finish by effleuraging the full leg x 1.

Feet

34) Take the stone from behind the right knee and use it to knead the sole of the right foot, thoroughly cover the sole of the foot. Knead up and down the instep with the stone to work on the reflex points for the spine (perform this movement slowly and check the pressure with the client).

Put the stone down and wring the foot and using the pad of your right thumb perform circular pressures on the Chakra part of the foot. Work from the Crown Chakra down the instep to the Root Chakra to close the Chakras down.

Repeat this procedure on the left foot.

CLOSING DOWN THE TREATMENT

To complete the treatment, begin at the head of the bed by the Crown Chakra and take the stone for the Crown Chakra, then take the stone for the Third Eye Chakra. Tap the two stones together twice to give the clear sound of the stones.

Now take the Throat Chakra stone and tap it twice with the stone from the Third Eye Chakra.

Move down all the Chakra stones in this way until they have all been removed from the body.

Pick the crystals up off the floor beneath the client's bed, again starting from the crown chakra and working down the root chakra.

It is very important that you now remove any remaining stones from the client and any on the bed before the client begins to move.

The treatment is now complete.

50% OFF FULL ACCESS

DON'T FORGET NOW YOU CAN USE A RANGE OF ONLINE LEARNING RESOURCES FOR JUST £10 (NORMAL RRP £20)

The Massage e-Learning Resource has been designed to enhance your learning experience

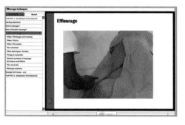

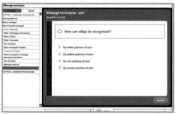

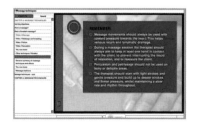

☐ Bring knowledge to life with videos of each technique as well as a full massage routine

☐ Manage your learning with step-by-step modules and integrated 'classroom' sessions

☐ Absorb information on key topics with interactive exercises and learning activities

To login to use these **e-learning resources**, visit **www.emspublishing.co.uk/massage** and follow the onscreen instructions

AN INTRODUCTORY GUIDE TO
Massage

10 Indian head massage

In Brief

In India massage has been used for thousands of years to treat mind and body. Indian head massage is a combination of ancient techniques and modern awareness of the importance of an holistic approach.

Learning objectives ●

The target knowledge of this chapter is:
● history of Indian Head massage
● benefits of Indian Head massage
● techniques of Indian Head massage
● scalp massage and using oils
● carrying out a treatment.

INDIAN HEAD MASSAGE

THE HISTORY OF INDIAN HEAD MASSAGE

In India Ayurvedic, or traditional, medicine is as important as orthodox medicine. It aims to treat the whole body in order to maintain a balance between the physical, mental and spiritual. Massage has always formed a central part of this. Indian families use massage on a daily basis both for relaxation and healing but also to maintain contact and enjoy the stress-reducing benefits of touch. From an early age children are taught to give head massage so that each family member can both give and receive treatment. At times of ritual, such as weddings and birth, massage has always been important. It is also common for men to receive a head massage when they visit the barber. Over the centuries, practitioners of alternative medicine have recognised the benefits of massage, particularly scalp massage, to relieve tension and stress. In the West the traditional scalp massage used in India has evolved to become Indian Head Massage – a treatment for the scalp, face, neck, shoulders and upper arms.

BENEFITS AND TECHNIQUES

What is Indian head massage?
Indian head massage uses and adapts classic Swedish massage techniques for treating the scalp, face, neck, shoulders and upper arms. It is extremely effective for treating stress because it works on the areas of the body most affected – the shoulders and upper back, neck and head. However, although the treatment focuses on the upper torso and head the effects are felt throughout the mind and body. It is performed on the client whilst clothed, which makes it very effective for short treatments and for treating clients who are uncomfortable about undressing. Oils which have traditionally been used to maintain strong, healthy, shiny hair can be used during the scalp massage but clothing prevents their use during other parts of the treatment.

What does it do?
Indian head massage has the following benefits:

- **skin:** encourages desquamation, and thus improves skin tone and colour.
- **skeletal system:** helps increase joint mobility and flexibility in shoulders, neck and arm. Reduces tension in tissues, making them more flexible which minimises the stress on bones and joints, reducing their need to overwork to compensate for muscles not working properly.
- **muscular system:** improved circulation helps remove waste, particularly lactic acid, from muscles, reducing aches and soreness; petrissage movements on neck and shoulders help reduce tension, stretch the tissues, increase flexibility, release tightness in overworked or tense muscles; stress reduction helps prevent stress-induced muscle spasm in back as well as shoulders and arms; reduction in inflammation or pain.
- **circulatory system:** improves circulation, thus improving the delivery of nutrients and oxygen and speeding up the removal of wastes and toxins; lowers blood pressure.
- **lymphatic system:** improves lymphatic circulation thus speeding up the removal of excess fluid and waste from cells, helping to reduce swelling and reducing the risk of infection through improved production and delivery of white blood cells.

- **nervous system:** reduces effects of stress thus facilitating sleep, reduces anxiety, slows down heart rate, improves breathing, releases physical and mental tension, promotes feelings of calm and well-being; helps unblock congestion throughout the body enabling improved neural communication; release of tension increases energy levels.

How do I do it?

The techniques used in Indian head massage are similar to those used in classic Swedish massage. There are five basic strokes.

Effleurage/Gentle stroking
What is it?

- preparatory and concluding stroke
- gentle and relaxing
- can be used superficially to relax or more deeply, applying more pressure, to stimulate the circulation and energise the client.

What does It do?

- prepares the client's mind and body for the deeper, firmer strokes
- warms the skin
- improves circulation, thereby helping to eliminate toxins from tissues and enabling them to work more efficiently
- relaxes and soothes nerve endings.

Petrissage/Kneading
What is it?

- kneading, squeezing stroke using whole hand or just fingers and thumbs which lifts tissues and muscles away from bones and joints, compresses them and then releases them.

What does it do?

- stretches the muscle fibres and tissues, thereby helping to reduce stiffness, inflexibility and tension
- encourages the elimination of waste and toxins from tissues
- improves circulation
- reduces nervous muscle spasm by helping release tension.

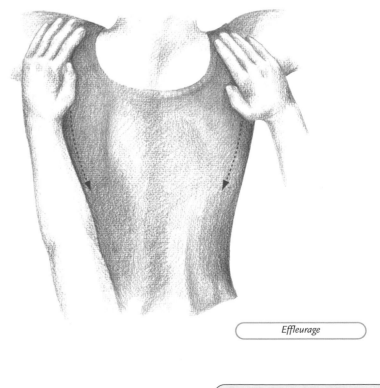

Effleurage

INDIAN HEAD MASSAGE

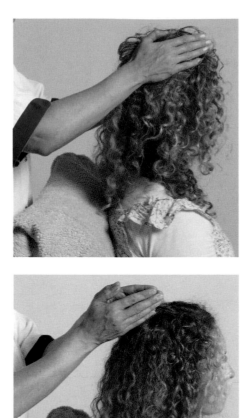

Champissage

Friction/Rubbing tissue against bone
What is it?
- a rubbing stroke, using either the whole hand or just the fingers, thumbs or palm of the hand, which compresses tissue against bone.

What does it do?
- improves circulation
- improves mobility by releasing tension in muscles
- when used on scalp encourages hair growth
- when used on skin helps desquamation thus improving skin tone and colour and encouraging cell regeneration.
- breaks down scar tissue and stimulates growth of new tissue.

Champissage (percussion)
What is it?
- movement using both hands together in a 'prayer' position in a rhythmic hacking movement
- can be used gently to relax or more firmly to energise and 'wake up' the body, particularly the nerves and muscles.

What does it do?
- stimulates the nerves
- improves the circulation
- energises the mind and body and provides a 'wake up'
- improves muscle tone.

Tabla
What is it?
- superficial tapping movement using the tops of the fingers or the heels of the hands
- can be used gently to relax or more firmly to energise and 'wake up' the body, particularly the nerves and muscles.

What does it do?
- stimulates the nerves
- improves the circulation
- energises the mind and body and provides a 'wake up'
- improves muscle tone.

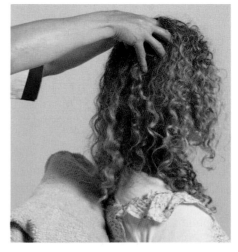

Friction

Pressure points

What is it?

- the application of pressure on specific points using fingertips and thumbs. These points, found along the 'meridians' of the body, release blocked 'energy'. Indian head massage often works on the 'chakras'.

What does it do?

- improves circulation
- encourages decongestion of the whole body thus boosting energy
- stimulates nerves.

What is scalp massage

Scalp massage uses specific massage techniques unique to this form of treatment. It stimulates the nerves and the blood supply to the scalp, using a combination of petrissage, friction, pressure and effleurage, and is the only part of Indian head massage where oils are used.

Why use oils?

Using oil conditions the scalp and the hair and adds to the relaxation. Tension sometimes causes hair loss and an oil massage can help stimulate hair growth. Oils are not always necessary or desired and their use will depend on the particular wishes/needs of the client. In some instances essential oils can be blended with a base oil for the scalp massage. The aromatic effects of the oils are enhanced by the fact that they are being used on the head, close to the olfactory tract and thus the oil molecules do not have to travel far. Also the client's breathing will usually be deeper and more relaxed and thus more effective at inhaling the smell.

Oils for a basic scalp massage are usually chosen because they moisturise the skin, condition the hair, stimulate hair growth and are neutral in scent. In India mustard oil, almond oil, coconut oil, sesame oil, and olive oil are traditionally used.

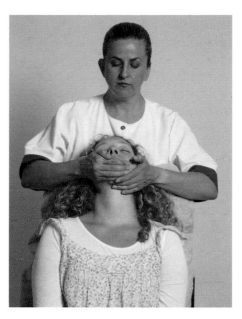

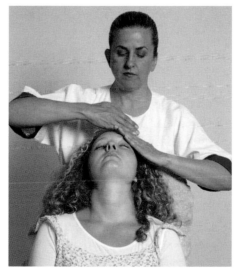

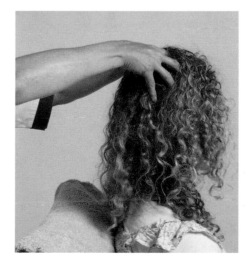

Mustard oil

Extracted from Yellow Mustard seeds. This oil is mainly used in north-west India. Mustard oil generates heat, making it popular for use in the cold winter months. It is particularly popular with males. Benefits include:

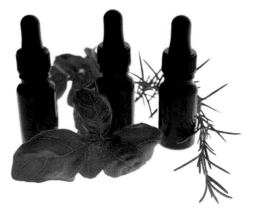

- stimulates circulation
- reduces pain and swelling
- soothes sore, tense muscles

Almond oil

A popular and easily obtainable oil in the West. Benefits include:
- good for mature skin and dry hair
- reduces muscular aches and pains
- calms the nerves

Coconut oil

Traditionally used by women as it has a sweet odour. Benefits include:
- lubricates dry skin and hair

Sesame oil

The most widely used oil in India. Benefits include:
- moisturises skin and hair
- reduces muscular aches and pains
- reduces swelling
- reduces stiffness
- reduces premature ageing

Olive oil

Benefits include:
- relieves the pain of arthritis

- relieves sore, tense muscles
- reduces swelling

However, both olive and mustard oil have strong scents and may thus be distracting rather than relaxing for some clients. Mustard oil can also be a skin irritant.

Which scalp conditions benefit from the use of oils?

- ### Alopecia

This is sudden and severe hair loss, usually caused by stress, shock, illness, chemotherapy and sometimes pregnancy. It is temporary and should not be confused with male pattern baldness, when hair loss is permanent. The bald patches are random and sometimes become red and/or scaly. An oil massage helps the client to relax, which can lessen the effect of the problem, conditions the scalp and stimulates hair growth. Clients should be encouraged to massage their scalp at home between treatments.

- ### Dandruff (pityriasis capitis/simplex)

Dandruff is a very common condition. It causes scales of dry skin to rub off the scalp into the hair. Often it can be treated with a shampoo. However, in more severe cases an oil massage will help by conditioning and reducing the dryness of the scalp.

- ### Eczema

Eczema causes the scalp to become dry, itchy, scaly and red. In some cases the scaly areas bleed. Oil massage can help twofold: since an attack of eczema is often caused by stress, the relaxing effects of the treatment can help reduce its recurrence; the oils used will help condition the scalp and reduce the itchiness. Olive oil is particularly good at treating eczema, but mustard oil should never be used. Common ailments that would benefit from Indian Head Massage include:

- Bell's Palsy
- headache
- temporo-mandibular joint tension (TMJ syndrome)
- tinnitus
- sycosis barbae (Barber's Itch)

You now know the techniques and benefits of Indian head massage. The next section explains the practicalities of carrying out a treatment.

One of the major practical benefits of Indian head massage is that it does not require the client to undress. This is very useful for two reasons: first, the nervous client or the client who is having a massage for the first time may feel uncomfortable about undressing and will feel reassured if this is not needed; second, the therapist needs very little equipment and can dispense with the changing facilities, towels or couch required for full body massage which means it is possible to work in a variety of environments, including the workplace.

CARRYING OUT A TREATMENT

What equipment is required?

The height of the client will affect the therapist's ability to reach their head and neck and the therapist needs to take this into account in order to prevent damage to themselves. A height-adjustable chair with proper lumbar support is the best type because it supports the client and also prevents the therapist from stooping. If a height-adjustable chair is not used, the therapist will need to use some form of bolster or cushion to adjust the client's height accordingly. If using oils for the scalp, a towel should be placed over the shoulders and a selection of base oils and, if required, essential oils should be easily accessible from the chair. (The same rule for all massages also applies to Indian head: keep at least one hand on the client once the treatment starts.)

What preparation is required for the client?

A consultation should be carried out to find out if there are any contraindications to Indian head massage. These are outlined in Chapter 5. However in addition note should be taken if the client has any of the following:
- pediculosis (lice)

- any contagious scalp conditions
- migraine
- nerves
- osteoporosis
- encephalitis
- meningitis
- poliomyelitis.

Clients should remove all obstacles to treatment such as jewellery, glasses and hair accessories and should be advised to wear something light through which it is possible to massage the shoulders and neck rather than thick jackets and jumpers. Long hair should be tied back until the scalp massage begins and then released. If necessary, hair should be brushed or combed to remove any products like hairspray, mousse, gel or wax.

Carrying out treatment

INDIAN HEAD MASSAGE

What preparation is required for the therapist?

The therapist should be able to reach the shoulders, neck, face and head of the client without overstretching. Adjust the height of the chair if necessary. Low shoes should be worn and long hair tied back. The therapist's posture and self-care is very important:

- keep back and legs straight but not rigid; the knees should be soft not locked
- adjust the position of the feet from standing to striding (see pp 60–61) when more pressure is needed
- relax the shoulders and upper back and avoid rolling shoulders up to the ears
- keep the head and neck aligned; avoid hanging the head and thus putting pressure on the neck and spine; lower the eyes rather than the whole head to look down and try to position the client so that it is not necessary to look down throughout the treatment
- keep the wrists straight and try to vary the movements to prevent repetitive strain injuries
- exercise the hands and wrists regularly
- keep hands scrupulously clean especially if using oils.

After treatment

Offer the client a glass of water and allow them a few minutes to 'wake up' from the deep relaxation. Explain that they may experience various reactions to treatment and that there is nothing to worry about. The body has been stimulated and relaxed and it is now adjusting to this by ridding itself of toxins and working on any problem areas that have been treated. Common reactions include:

- increased desire to urinate
- intensified emotional reactions
- tiredness
- lightheadedness
- aching muscles
- increase in production of mucous from the nasal passages
- healing crisis where symptoms become worse for a few hours before they begin to improve.

You now know what Indian head Massage is, what it does, which techniques are required and how to carry out a treatment.

Client Consultation Form – Indian Head massage

College Name: Indian Head Massage School
College Number: 0002
Student Name: Mary Panton
Student Number: A12345
Date: 15th October

Client Name: Tim
Address: On file

Profession: IT
Tel. No: Day On file
Eve On file

PERSONAL DETAILS

Age group: ☐ Under 20 ☐ 20–30 ☐ 30–40 ☑ 40–50 ☐ 50–60 ☐ 60+
Lifestyle: ☐ Active ☑ Sedentary
Last visit to the doctor: ☐ September
GP Address: On file
No. of children (if applicable): 0
Date of last period (if applicable): n/a

CONTRAINDICATIONS REQUIRING MEDICAL PERMISSION – in circumstances where medical permission cannot be obtained clients must give their informed consent in writing prior to treatment (select where/if appropriate):

☐ Cardiovascular conditions (thrombosis, phlebitis, hypertension
☐ Haemophilia
☐ Any condition already being treated by a GP or another complementary practitioner
☐ Medical oedema
☐ Osteoporosis
☐ Arthritis
☐ Nervous/Psychotic conditions
☐ Epilepsy
☐ Recent operations
☐ Diabetes
☐ Asthma

☐ Any dysfunction of the nervous system (e.g. Multiple sclerosis, Parkinson's disease, Motor neurone disease)
☐ Trapped/Pinched nerve (e.g. sciatica)
☐ Inflamed nerve
☐ Cancer
☐ Postural deformities
☐ Spastic conditions
☐ Whiplash
☐ Slipped disc
☐ Undiagnosed pain
☐ When taking prescribed medication
☐ Acute rheumatism

CONTRAINDICTIONS THAT RESTRICT TREATMENT (select where/if appropriate):

☐ Fever
☐ Contagious or infectious diseases
☐ Under the influence of recreational drugs or alcohol
☐ Diarrhoea and vomiting
☐ Pediculosis Capitis (head lice)
☐ Conjunctivitis
☐ Sycosis barbae
☐ Skin diseases
☐ Undiagnosed lumps and bumps
☐ Localised swelling
☐ Inflammation
☐ Cuts
☐ Bruises
☐ Abrasions
☐ Myalgic Encephalomyelitis (chronic fatigue syndrome)
☐ Psoriasis

☐ Scar tissues (2 years for major operation and 6 months for a small scar)
☐ Sunburn
☐ Hormonal implants
☐ Recent fractures (minimum 3 months)
☐ Cervical spondylitis
☐ After a heavy meal
☐ Anaphylaxis
☐ Vertigo
☐ Adhesive capsulitis
☐ Bells Palsy
☐ Tinnitus
☐ Migraine
☐ Earache
☐ Headaches

WRITTEN PERMISSION REQUIRED BY:

☐ GP/Specialist ☐ Informed consent
Either of which should be attached to the consultation form.

PERSONAL INFORMATION (select if/where appropriate):

Muscular/Skeletal problems: ☑ Back ☑ Aches/Pain ☐ Stiff joints ☑ Headaches

Digestive problems: ☐ Constipation ☑ Bloating ☐ Liver/Gall bladder ☐ Stomach

Circulation: ☐ Heart ☑ Blood pressure ☐ Fluid retention ☐ Tired legs ☐ Varicose veins
☐ Cellulite ☐ Kidney problems ☐ Cold hands and feet ☐ Borderline low blood pressure 110/80

Gynaecological: ☐ Irregular periods ☐ P.M.T ☐ Menopause ☐ H.R.T ☐ Pill ☐ Coil
Other: _____

Nervous system: ☐ Migraine ☐ Tension ☑ Stress ☑ Depression

Immune system: ☐ Prone to infections ☐ Sore throats ☐ Colds ☐ Chest ☐ Sinuses

Regular antibiotic/medication taken? ☐ Yes ☑ No
If yes, which ones: _____

Herbal remedies taken? ☐ Yes ☑ No
If yes, which ones: _____

Ability to relax: ☑ Good ☐ Moderate ☐ Poor

Sleep patterns: ☑ Good ☐ Poor ☐ Average No. of hours 8

Do you see natural daylight in your workplace? ☐ Yes ☑ No

Do you work at a computer? ☑ Yes ☐ No If yes how many hours 10

Do you eat regular meals? ☑ Yes ☐ No

Do you eat in a hurry? ☑ Yes ☐ No

Do you take any food/vitamin supplements? ☐ Yes ☑ No
If yes, which ones: _____

How many portions of each of these items does your diet contain per day?
Fresh fruit: 2 Fresh vegetables: 3 Protein: 3 source? Meat, chicken
Dairy produce: 3 Sweet things: 3 Added salt: 1 Added sugar: 3

How many units of these drinks do you consume per day?
Tea: 3 Coffee: 0 Fruit juice: 2 Water: 4 Soft drinks: 0 Others: 0

Do you suffer from food allergies? ☐ Yes ☑ No Bingeing? ☐ Yes ☑ No
Overeating? ☐ Yes ☑ No

Do you smoke? ☑ No ☐ Yes How many per day?

Do you drink alcohol? ☐ No ☑ Yes How many units per day? 1

Do you exercise? ☑ None ☐ Occasional ☐ Irregular ☐ Regular
Types: _____

What is your skin type? ☐ Dry ☐ Oil ☑ Combination ☐ Sensitive ☐ Dehydrated

Do you suffer/have you suffered from: ☐ Dermatitis ☐ Acne ☐ Eczema ☐ Psoriasis
☐ Allergies ☐ Hay Fever ☐ Asthma ☐ Skin cancer

Stress level: 1–10 (10 being the highest)
At work 4   At home 3

Reason for treatment: To help alleviate back and neck pain due to poor posture and frequent head
aches
_____
_____
_____
_____
_____
_____

CLIENT PROFILE

Tim is a 45 year old divorced man who is self employed working in IT. He works from home which often means he can go for a couple of days without going out. He loves his job but sometimes finds it stressful when he is unsure where his next account is coming from. He meets friends in the pub three times a week when he drinks beer. He cooks his own food but has a sweet tooth and often eats too much of the wrong things and he always eats in a hurry and often feels bloated. He is very tall and suffers from kyphosis through bad posture which leads to ongoing back and neck pain with headaches almost daily. He rarely exercises and sometime feels depressed

TREATMENT 1

Treatment plan
To give Tim a course of three Indian Head Massages at weekly intervals concentrating on back, neck, shoulders and scalp. He was happy for me to use olive oil on his scalp for its anti-inflammatory properties

Details of how the client felt during the treatment:
As expected Tim held a huge amount of tension in his neck and shoulders and at the beginning of the massage his back felt stiff and rigid. Because of this I added extra effleurage, kneading and champissage over his upper back and shoulders. He wanted to talk but I suggested that he thought about slowing and deepening his breathing to aid his relaxation. I could tell he was finding it hard to relax but when I began massaging his scalp using a small amount of olive oil I felt him suddenly relax. He stayed relaxed until the end of the massage

Details of how the client felt after the treatment:
Tim commented that initially he found it hard to relax even though he was Enjoying the massage but once I began to massage his scalp he absolutely adored it and wished he had discovered Indian Head massage years ago. He could not believe how different his neck and head now felt

Details of home care advice given:
I advised Tim to go home and relax, drink plenty of water and have a light evening meal. As Tim had not had an Indian Head massage before I explained the possible side effects to the treatment and told him not to worry if he did feel a little under the weather and if that happened he should drink more water and that it shouldn't last longer than 24 hours. I recommended that Tim should go out for a walk at least once a day as daylight and exercise help with mood and aid relaxation.
I said he should be aware of his posture while sitting at the computer. He said he knew he sat very badly but had never bothered to do anything about it.
I told him that if he ate his food slowly he might find the bloating goes away

Reflective practice:
I found Tim hard to massage as the tension in his back and neck was so great he found it difficult to sit up correctly and I found I was leaning forward to compensate. I also need a slightly larger support for his head during the face massage

INDIAN HEAD MASSAGE

TREATMENT 2

Tim had a bad headache after his first treatment which lasted until he woke the next morning. He asked if he was likely to have another bad headache after today's treatment which I said was less likely. Tim said his shoulders felt so much better but his neck was still tight and stiff and he had still be getting headaches though they were not as bad. He was really looking forward to today's massage where again I will concentrate on his back, neck, shoulders and scalp.

Details of how the client felt during the treatment:

Tim still had a lot of tension in his upper back but today he closed his eyes, focused on his breathing and relaxed straight away. I used deeper effleurage, kneading and frictions than last week to try and alleviate as much tension as I could. I used olive oil again in the scalp massage as Tim commented on how nice his hair felt after he had washed it

Details of how the client felt after the treatment:

Again Tim was very relaxed and he commented that this time he relaxed right from the start of the massage

Details of homecare advice given:

Tim remembered the previous aftercare advice and said he will drink more water for the rest of the day.

During the week he had gone for a short walk almost every morning and said he felt happier than he had for a while

Tim was also trying to improve his posture while at the computer but finding it hard

He was forgetting to eat slower. I asked him where he ate his meals and he said in front of his computer. So I suggested he sat at a table while he ate and then he might remember to eat slowly.

Reflective practice:

I still found it hard to maintain good posture while massaging Tim but the larger support helped when I was massaging his face. I was happy with the pressure I was using and felt that my champissage had improved since the last treatment

TREATMENT 3

Tim did not have a headache after last weeks massage and said he felt wonderful for at least four days afterwards but he is still getting headaches most days. Tim is looking forward to today's Indian Head massage. I will again focus on the problem areas.

Details of how the client felt during the treatment:

I used a deeper pressure again this week as it seemed to make such a difference to how Tim felt during the week. Although there was still a lot of tension in his upper back and neck it did seem a little more pliable than the previous weeks.

Details of how the client felt after the treatment:

Tim again felt wonderful and was very complementary about my massage. He felt the pressure was firmer than the week before which he really liked.

Details of home care advice given:

Tim was still walking almost every day and he said again how much better he felt for it.

He was still trying to improve his posture while sitting in front of the computer. He was thinking about investing in a better chair.
He was still eating in front of the computer and still in a hurry
I recommended that because of the headaches and neck pain that it might be a good idea to go and see a chiropractor or osteopath as it was possible is his neck might need an adjustment

Reflective practice:

Tim was so happy with his Indian Head massages he has done a lot for my confidence and I think that helped me give him a firmer massage this week. I am also finding the routine much easier to remember now and because of that I think my massage and posture has improved nicely

Overall conclusion of the case study:

Tim was very pleased with the outcome. His neck and back felt better than it had in years and although he was still getting headaches they were not as bad as before. He felt going out every day had made such a difference to the way he felt mentally. He also said he will bear in mind that he should be eating his food slower and if he does remember to do that he will see if that makes a difference to his bloating. Tim said he will go and see the chiropractor I recommended and he also would like to continue having Indian Head massages at least fortnightly.

INDIAN HEAD MASSAGE ROUTINE

Shoulders and Arms

Make the client comfortable, ensuring that their feet are flat on the floor and their hands/arms are in an open but comfortable position. Stand behind the client and place you hands on their shoulders. Take 3 deep breaths in and out to centre yourself before beginning the routine. Ask the client to do the same.

1) Full effleurage over the whole area to be worked – covering trapezius, rhomboids and deltoids – three times

2) Using anti clockwise circles rub the whole area to be worked on with a light pressure one side, then the other, supporting the opposite shoulder – three times.

3) Heel rub around the border of the scapula in a 'C' shape – three times, one side then the other, covering part of latissimus dorsi, teres major, teres minor, the rhomboids, part of erector spinae, infraspinalis, the edge of supraspinalis, trapezius and the deltoid.

4) Finger pad friction around the border of the scapula in a 'C' shape as before – three times, one side then the other

5) Thumb pushes from shoulder to neck – working from the edge of the trapezius into the centre, gently squeezing from the top of the shoulder working towards the neck. Slide out and repeat 3 times.

6) Finger pulls – anchor thumb at back and draw up and over working from top of shoulder into neck – three times.

7) Place one hand either side of client's upper arms, then roll the heel of the hand around the arm to meet the fingers, but without pinching – three times.

8) Link the fingers of both hands and then facing the shoulder, apply gentle pressure as you squeeze and lift the tissues, release then repeat this movement working down over the deltoid, biceps and triceps to the elbow. Do not pinch the tissues. Slide back to the deltoid to start again – three times.

9) Smooth down with the forearms to the elbow x 3, sliding back up to begin again

10) Slide one hand down either side of the client, from deltoid to elbow. Holding under the elbow, keeping the arms close to the body, lift the arms upwards ensuring client comfort throughout and working within client limitations. Then, return them to the starting position –three times.

11) Champissage - Hold the hands as if praying, keeping fingers relaxed. Fingertips and the heels of the hands should be touching. Begin to hack gently over the area following the 'C' shape around the base of the scapula, working up to and along the trapezius to the edge of the shoulder. Repeat each side, three times

12) Using both hands effleurage over the scapula, deltoids & trapezius to finish - three times.

Neck
Support the client's head throughout this part of the routine.

1) Place hands on occipital and frontal areas. Move the client's head gently to the front and then the back to release tension in the neck – three times.

2) Supporting the frontal area with one hand, then slide down the contours of the neck using the thumb & fingers with a medium pressure – three times.

3) Supporting the frontal area with one hand, knead down neck three times

4) Thumb pushes from back of neck to front, working from the base of the neck up to the ear – three times. Follow in the same pattern with vibrations using the fingertips.

5) Incline the head and support, resting the arm on the client's shoulder and supporting with the hand – friction up the neck to the occipital area, slide back down. Repeat three times.

6) Incline head and stretch neck, smoothing back of the neck with the forearm – three times each side.

7) Smooth over neck with the hand – three times

Head and Scalp
1) By placing hands on the top of the head just take a deep breath & relax.

2) Begin to stroke over the head lightly, using one hand at a time.

3) Supporting with one hand, use the ball of the hand to rub lightly over the head – three times. Repeat on other side.

4) Support the head with one hand and then begin to move the other hand over the scalp with a firm pressure until one side of scalp is covered, hairline to occipital. Change hands and repeat.

5) Using fingertips, ruffle through the hair front to back.

6) Tabla – use the fingertips to tap all over the client's scalp to stimulate the circulation. Cover the whole scalp.

7) Pulling through the hair, one hand and then the other. Then gently tug on the client's hair.

8) Place one hand either side of the scalp, then squeeze hands together and lift the scalp gently. Repeat three times then do the same with hands on the occipital and frontal areas – three times

9) Vibrate fingers all over scalp. Comb through hair with fingers to finish.

Face
Sanitise hands before moving onto the face. Place appropriate covered support behind the client and ask them to lean back slightly within their range of comfort.

1) Face brace to cover the skin – three times

2) Stroking over the brow – three times each side

3) Apply pressure along points above the inner eyebrow using the tips of

INDIAN HEAD MASSAGE

the 4th finger (ring), working out to the side, to the temporal area – three times.

4) Tap over the face from jaw to forehead gently and rapidly with the fingertips – three times to cover the whole face in a continual movement.

5) Glide down then sweep fingers along jaw line from the centre towards the ears – alternate sides – three times

6) Glide up and apply pressure underneath the cheekbones using the tip of the 4th finger working from either side of the nose out to the anterior auricular nodes – three times.

7) Stroking under the eyes from the sides of the nose out – very gently, using alternate fingertips – 4th finger. The skin must not move.

8) Rotating the fingertip apply pressure gently to finger circle on the temples – three times.

9) Move the hands to the ears and knead around the edge of the ears, down and back up – three times.

10) Stroking through the hair to finish.

Chakra balancing may also be performed over the throat, brow and crown chakras to complete the treatment if the client is receptive.

Ensure the client's head is brought back to the centre gently. Remove the support and in a gentle and calming voice suggest your client comes back into focus in their own time. Offer them a them a glass of water. Once they are ready, go through after and home care advice. As Indian head massage can have dramatic effects, help them to stand up if necessary and escort them from the treatment room.

11 Sports massage

In Brief

Sports massage combines the use of Swedish massage with additional more intensive techniques, for the prevention and treatment of sports injuries. The first part of this chapter explains what sports massage is, the second explains how to apply it.*

NB Sports massage therapy is a complex and wide-ranging subject. Within the remit of an introductory guide to massage it is not possible to cover all aspects of this therapy. This chapter therefore offers an introduction to the practical uses and benefits of sports massage, and not a detailed theoretical approach.

Learning objectives ●

The target knowledge of this chapter is:
- definition of sports massage
- benefits of sports massage
- advanced techniques
- when to use sports massage
- assessing the client and carrying out treatment
- how exercise affects the body: special considerations specific to sports massage
- special dietary considerations specific to sports massage

WHAT IS SPORTS MASSAGE?

Sports massage is the use of massage for the treatment and prevention of sports injuries. It can be used as part of a training programme to help prevent injury, as part of a rehabilitation programme to treat injury, as part of a warm-up for an event and as part of the wind-down after the event.

and assists body systems in functioning at their optimum level. Sports massage also has more specific effects and benefits:

- speeds up the healing of damaged or overworked tissue and muscles thus reduces recovery time and allows a sports person to regain their health and performance
- increases fitness capabilities and performance potential
- prevents future injury by identifying and treating current muscle weakness, tiredness and problem areas
- post-event massage helps clear out waste and toxins, e.g. lactic acid from muscles, reducing stiffness and enabling a faster recovery than post-event rest
- massage helps break up adhesions that can develop between the fascia of different muscles, thus improving muscle suppleness and mobility
- enables muscles and joints to heal faster after injury
- improves flexibility
- peak performance can be reached faster and, once reached, sustained over longer periods.

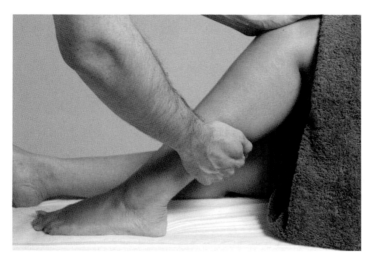

What does it do?

Sports massage, like other forms of massage, helps improve the suppleness and flexibility of muscles and joints. It improves lymph and blood circulation

ADVANCED TECHNIQUES

Sports massage combines classic Swedish massage movements such as effleurage with other, more advanced techniques such as lymphatic drainage, compression, frictioning, neuro-muscular technique, muscle energy technique, soft tissue release and connective tissue massage.

Effleurage and petrissage

Sports massage effleurage (stroking) is very similar to effleurage used in other forms of massage. However, in addition to traditional effleurage which is performed using the palms, it may

involve the use of the lower arm to apply deeper pressure strokes over larger areas. Petrissage in sports massage relies on the elbow, fist or heel of the hand (the lower part of the palm) to apply the classic kneading movements and deeper pressure to the body.

Lymphatic drainage massage

The lymphatic system is a secondary circulation that helps the circulatory system, the function of which is to drain the tissue spaces of the body of excess fluid. It collects toxins and excess fluid from the cells and tissues, filters off bacteria, produces antibodies and returns the filtered fluid and antibodies to the circulatory system. Lymphatic drainage massage can help the action of the lymphatic system, encouraging the removal of toxins and boosting the immune system. It is useful for treating fluid retention or oedema (swelling). Manual lymphatic drainage uses:

- gentle, pumping movements in the direction of the lymph nodes
- light pressure because many lymph vessels are near the surface of the skin and firm or deep pressure is thought to prevent lymph movement.

See Chapter 7 for more information on lymphatic drainage massage.

Kneading to the gastrocnemius

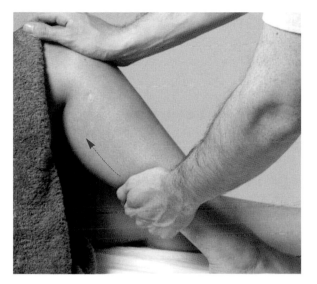

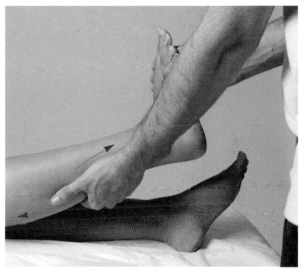

Compression

Compression is the application of pressure to the body using the heel of the hand (base of the palm) or the fist to push the muscle tissue against the bone. Like squeezing, compression has a pumping effect, assisting circulation. The therapist should begin pressing at the insertion of the muscle and move along to its origin. It is generally used longitudinally, along the length of a muscle but it can also be used transversally, as with cross-fibre frictions, to help ease stiffness out of a muscle and make it more supple.

Deep friction (also known as cross-fibre friction)

Deep friction is a variant of the friction technique described in Chapter 3. The pads of the thumb(s) and the tips of the fingers or elbows are placed on the

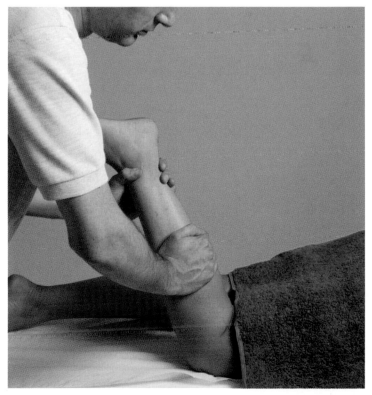

surface of the skin and used to apply firm pressure. The therapist then rubs the skin immediately below the fingers and thumbs, thus moving the surface (subcutaneous) layer of tissue against the deeper layer of tissue. However, whereas friction is usually used along the length of the muscle, cross-fibre works across the muscle (hence the name). This helps to stretch the muscle fibres and release tension. It also allows the therapist to work close to a damaged or inflamed area without touching it because working on one section of muscle helps stretch the rest of the muscle. It is a focused technique generally used to work on a small area. The client may feel discomfort at the start of the friction but the effect should be one of heat and subsequent release, not pain. The therapist may suggest that the client use deep breathing or relaxation techniques to ensure that they do not tense up during the treatment, which would be counterproductive. Working very closely with the muscles helps to break down any local 'knottiness', lumpiness or adhesions and thus improves muscle function, elasticity and efficiency.

Neuromuscular Technique

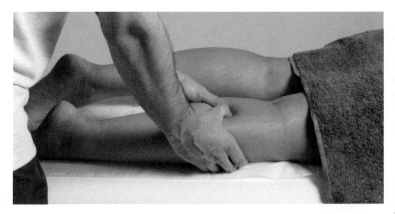

(NMT)

Neuromuscular technique is a form of friction. However, in this case instead of moving the thumb and/or fingers over an

area the digit is held in place over a sore point and pressure is gradually increased up to the limits of the client's pain threshold. It is very important to stress to the client that their feedback is vital so that further damage is not caused. The pressure should be maintained until the pain begins to decrease. In some instances the thumb or finger in use can be circled on the sore area. Deep pressure on a damaged area helps provoke a reflex in the nervous system which helps the muscles relax in the area treated.

Muscle Energy Technique (MET)

Muscle energy technique is a variety of techniques that involve restricted or resistive movement to stretch muscles. These movements require the client to resist the therapist's movements of the joints. The therapist stretches the muscles out until the resistance is felt and before pain and discomfort are felt. Once at that point, the patient should be asked to push gently against the therapist's hold for 5–10 seconds and then released. The therapist will now find further stretching can be achieved without resistance therefore increasing movement. This procedure can be repeated 2–3 times.

Soft Tissue Release (STR)

Soft tissue release combines pressure and movement. Pressure is applied to the area with the muscle relaxed or in shortened position. The muscle is stretched causing the muscle fibres to lengthen and stretch, releasing adhesions or 'stickiness'.

Connective Tissue Massage (CTM)

This is not a massage as such but a form of stretching to release the fluids trapped within the connective tissue between the muscle fibres. Using CTM techniques any adhesions in the superficial connective tissue layers are broken up and relaxed through reflexes.

No massage medium is used as it only involves stretching using the tips and pads of the fingers, particularly the middle finger. The pressure is dependant upon the angle of the fingers and the depth of the problem area.

For short distances, the middle finger moves along the area taking up the loose skin ensuring a stretching effect is achieved before releasing, allowing the skin to return. For longer distances, more fingers can be used with longer strokes incorporated before releasing.

Pressure can be applied in both directions ensuring rhythm and pressure is constant. Strokes can be repeated between three and ten times to allow for correct skin reaction.

CTM is useful in sports massage when a patient has extremely tender and tight muscles; by releasing the superficial tension the muscle can be softened therefore allowing further massage treatment to proceed.

You now know what sports massage is and the advanced techniques it requires. The next section explains how and when to use it.

USING SPORTS MASSAGE

Which techniques should I use?

The techniques used depend on the client's condition and needs. The five main uses of sports massage — pre-event, post-event, between-event, preventative and corrective — all require a particular treatment.

Pre-event – what is it?

Pre-event massage is used before a sporting event or performance. Its purpose is to stimulate the body (in particular the muscle groups that are most important to the event) and mind of the athlete in order that he or she can perform to their full capacity. It should stimulate the circulation so that all the cells of the body have enough oxygen and nutrients to work at their optimum level and that waste, particularly lactic acid, is rapidly removed and does not build up causing stiffness or cramp. Local circulation will also be stimulated, causing vasodilation and warming the skin and local tissues of the treatment area. Finally, pre-event massage helps prepare the muscular and nervous systems for a co-ordinated response to the athlete's demands. It is part of the warm-up, not a replacement for it.

Which techniques are used?

Providing high stimulation is required, techniques such as petrissage, compression and percussion (hacking and cupping; see Chapter 3), should be used in conjunction with an oil medium. However, relaxation *before* an event may also be necessary to combat nervousness. The therapist should aim for maximum stimulation of the muscles, using brisk, rapid strokes and though petrissage is an integral part of this treatment it should not be used for too long because it may induce relaxation instead of the required invigoration. In addition, the therapist should aim to treat the whole body without working on one area for too long to prevent over-working and fatiguing one section and to keep the athlete warm. The therapist should avoid using relaxing strokes, unless the athlete is tense about the event in which case some slower strokes can be used to lessen the anxiety. Pre-event massage treatment should only be given if the athlete has previously been treated with massage during training or rehabilitation because the massage may disrupt the athlete's performance if he or she is not used to it.

Why use it?

Pre-event massage stimulates the circulation and helps the body to work at its optimum level. Focusing on the specific muscles involved optimises muscle performance and flexibility. It stimulates the mind and body preparing it for the workout ahead.

Post-event massage – what is it?

Post-event massage is used after a sporting event or performance. Treatment should take place as soon as possible after the event, preferably in the first two hours. Most sports, particularly contact sports, will cause some microtrauma to the body, even if only to the skin and superficial tissues. Post-event massage helps to start the healing process required to prevent these microtraumas from becoming problematic. It cleanses the body, ridding it of the waste built up in the muscles during the event and facilitates relaxation and efficient recovery.

Which techniques are used?

Post-event massage should concentrate on compression, effleurage, connective tissue massage and petrissage. These are relaxing and cleansing strokes, helping the body to remove toxins. Superficial and deep effleurage help to push the waste and lactic acid build-up out of the muscles and into the blood and lymph circulation to be removed. Petrissage also helps remove waste as well as focussing on stiff or sore areas, reducing fatigue and soreness and making stiff muscles more supple. Light pressure should be used to prevent further damage to areas overworked or traumatised by exertion and strokes should be soothing and rhythmic both to maintain stimulation to the blood and lymphatic circulation as the athlete cools down as well as to prevent fluid collecting in vessels.

1. Mark Beck,
The Theory and Practice of Therapeutic Massage, Tarrytown, NY: Milady, 1988. Page 363

Why use it?

Post-event massage enables a rapid and safe cooling down from the exertion of sport. It may also help to reduce or prevent swelling and help stretch and relax tense muscle fibres. Furthermore, research has proved that post-event massage is three to four times more effective than rest as a way of recovering from muscle fatigue.[1] This is because it stimulates the lymph and blood circulation which helps to remove any lactic acid build-up, thereby reducing muscle fatigue and stiffness. In turn this helps prevent future injury by enabling the muscles to rest properly and heal faster. It can therefore help an athlete to recover from an event and resume their training schedule much more quickly.

Between-event massage – what is it?

This type of massage is used in multiple event situations such as knock-out competitions or pentathlons. It aims to combine both pre-and post-event techniques, thus treating any damage or fatigue as well as preparing the body for the next event.

Why use it?

Between-event massage can speed up the recovery from the preceding event allowing the body to prepare itself more rapidly for the next. It helps to remove any lactic acid build-up, which thus enables efficient muscle function and helps reduce any swelling or complication of any microtrauma suffered.

Preventative massage – what is it?

Preventative massage is the most useful form of sports massage. It forms part of an athlete's training programme and is used to improve general performance and to pinpoint and protect problem areas.

Which techniques are used?

Preventative massage treatment focuses on an overall treatment, combining petrissage, effleurage, percussion, connective tissue massage and friction, as well as more localised treatment for those areas most used by the athlete. For example, a runner would be treated with a general massage with particular focus on the legs using friction and cross-fibre frictions to treat any tight, sore or sticky muscle fibres.

Why use it?

Preventative massage improves blood and lymph circulation, thus improving the delivery of nutrients and oxygen and the removal of waste and carbon dioxide from every cell. This enables muscles to work more efficiently which in turn prevents muscle damage. Massage makes muscles more supple and mobile, reduces stiffness and loosens adhesions thus improving general flexibility and muscle tone, enhancing performance and helping to prevent injury. Finally, preventative massage used as part of training can help identify muscle problems at an early stage, thus reducing the likelihood of performance being affected.

Corrective massage – what is it?

Corrective massage is used as a treatment for injuries. It is the most focused of the four treatments because it pinpoints problem areas, such as past injuries, current injuries or weak spots and those muscle groups most in use and therefore most likely to be damaged.

Which techniques are used?

Frictions, including cross-fibre frictions, compression, petrissage, neuro-muscular technique and vibrations are most useful. Effleurage is more relaxing and should only be used at the beginning and end of treatment, rather than for the

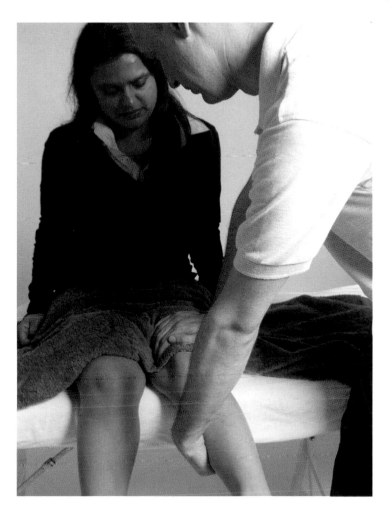

Muscle strength testing

more intense work. Pain is an inevitable part of treating damaged tissue but the therapist should not continue to work an area if the discomfort felt is causing the client to tense up. Try applying gentle pressure to a painful area for a few seconds; if the pain doesn't worsen or lessens, then it is generally safe to work the area but otherwise it should be avoided and the client referred to a GP before treatment. This is also a general pre-massage gauge.

Why use it?

Corrective massage enables faster healing of, and recovery from, injuries.

You now know the different techniques and approaches required for the different types of sports massage. The next section explains how to assess the client's needs and carry out treatment.

SPORTS MASSAGE

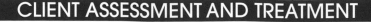

CLIENT ASSESSMENT AND TREATMENT

How do I find out where the problems are and what to treat?

For the first massage treatment, the therapist will need to palpate (feel) the client's muscles to look for problem areas, lumpiness, tightness and adhesions. Any pain felt is an indicator of injury or damage to a muscle. Tightness or lumpiness indicates tension or that the muscle has not healed properly after a previous injury. Palpation generally reveals problem areas in superficial muscles; deep muscles are usually inaccessible.

What is palpation?

Palpation is the method used to assess muscles and/or the degree of swelling or damage. Very simply, it is the process of using the palms of the hand (or fingertips for smaller or more tender areas) to touch the different muscles and parts of the body in order to determine their condition. The process is two-way – as the therapist touches the different areas of the body the client needs to explain whether there is any pain or discomfort in the various muscles, so that the therapist can assess the muscle in terms of both how it feels to the touch and how the client feels when it is touched. Generally, the pressure used will depend on the area being assessed – a thigh for example contains many more layers of muscle than a hand and therefore requires more pressure to access the deeper layers. However, sometimes damage is too deep to be felt by the therapist's hands. For assessment of deeper areas, the non-working hand should be used for support because sometimes a reflex action in a muscle other than the one being palpated can suggest a problem. Tension in superficial muscles may also be caused by a problem in a deeper layer of muscle.

Palpation should be carried out slowly, to ensure that the assessment is thorough. The pressure used should be light at the start then gradually increased to prevent any muscle tension developing or causing discomfort to the client. This is especially important on areas that are obviously inflamed or that the client has cited as a problem. Throughout the palpation, the therapist should pay attention to all client feedback, both verbal and physical.

What does a healthy muscle feel like?

Healthy muscles should be smooth, without lumps, spasm or tightness, easy to move and should not hurt when deep effleurage is used. The tendons should be firm but not stiff.

What does a problem area feel like?

Problem areas fall into several categories. When assessing muscles look for the following:

- **tension:** muscle fibres will be difficult to move and not very flexible
- **adhesions:** after injury or inflammation, tissue-making cells, known as fibroblasts, rush to the area and start mending the damage with collagen fibres. In some instances, especially if the muscle remained tense after the injury or healing was not completed properly the new tissue does not receive enough oxygen and nutrients and becomes 'sticky' and inflexible, like scar tissue, and the muscle fibres stick together. In some instances the fibres develop between different muscle fascias sticking them together. As a result the muscles will not be as efficient, other local muscles, bones and joints will adjust and overwork to compensate for the

weakness of the damaged area and the problem, instead of being treated, will become part of the body's structure. Adhesions feel much less smooth than normal tissue.

- **previous injury:** scar tissue is not as mobile or as pliable as normal tissue. Old scar tissue feels lumpy and solid, with little or no flexibility. More recent scar tissue will feel firm with a little flexibility. Wherever damage has occurred the muscles will be rather stiff and inflexible.
- **fatty nodules:** these occur close to the skin's surface and feel lumpy to the touch
- **swelling (oedema):** indicates recent injury or an injury that has not healed properly. The lymph fluid is the body's protection for a damaged area, allowing it to concentrate on sorting out the problem. Swelling can be detected by pressing with a finger on an area that appears swollen then removing the finger: if the finger leaves a white mark in the area oedema is present. Also the affected area will feel watery and full of fluid. Extremely swollen areas will be firmer, even solid, relatively immobile and painful due to the excess fluid pressure on the sensory nerves.
- **painful areas:** try and work out if the pain is caused by any of the above. If not, and if the client themself was unaware of the problem before the massage refer them to a GP before continuing with treatment.
- **inflammation:** look for redness, heat and pain. Superficial inflammation can be treated by working on other areas near the problem. For example, if the inflammation is at one end of a muscle, working the belly and other end will stretch the muscle in the affected area without pain and help it to heal.
- **tear in muscle:** look for a dip or hole in the muscle contour where the fibres

are no longer close together. If this occurs, advise client to seek medical attention.

The causes and effects of sports injuries

It is important for therapists to know the causes of sports injuries so that they can tailor the treatment to the actual problem. Consultation and palpation are just as important as treatment because they allow the therapist to find out, both verbally and physically the most likely assessment and thus treatment for a problem.

Compresses

A compress is a piece of material that has been soaked in water and is then placed over an affected part of the body and held in place for a period of time.
Both hot and cold compresses can be used: hot compresses are more useful for muscular aches and pains, earaches and toothaches whereas cold compresses are better for joint sprains and headaches. Both hot and cold compresses may be used to ease painful joints, aching muscles or cool a fevered brow.

Using Compresses

To make a compress:
1. fill a bowl with 100mls of hot or cold water
2. soak a piece of material (e.g. a flannel or unmedicated gauze) in the bowl of water
3. squeeze out the excess water and place the material over the affected area
4. cover with cling film to hold the material in place and leave for approximately two hours
5. the compress will soon cool down/warm up. Repeat the process as long as is necessary or desired

The following table lists the most common sports injuries and their effects.

Injury	Cause	Effects
Adhesive capsulitis (frozen shoulder)	Wrenched shoulder, overuse, may follow injury to disc in the neck	Pain and restriction of movement in the shoulder joint.
Calcaneal bursitis	Inflammation of the bursa between the calcaneum and the insertion of the Achilles tendon possibly due to a strain or ill fitting shoes.	Back of the heel feels tender and bruised, no pain when contracting the tendon e.g. standing on or pointing the toes.
Carpal Tunnel Syndrome	Long standing compression found in cycling or from repeated blows in racquet and batting sports.	Acute inflammation of the tendons, causing pressure on the median nerve. Persistent dull ache in thumb and first two fingers, usually worse at night. Lack of grip in the hand.
Chondromalacia patella	Due to repeated minor impacts or occasional major impacts on the knee joint. Also prolonged static or dynamic load on the knee joint during sports like sailing, downhill skiing and weight lifting.	Pain in knee when walking up and down stairs and hills with more pain felt going down
Chronic muscle fatigue	Overuse of muscle fibres which could become irritated and inflamed causing tightness.	Tight muscle causes the athlete to under perform, slows down rate of improvement and could result in injury.
Concussion	Blow to the head – when athlete collides with another and hits his or her head, falls from a height, or sustains a blow on the jaw.	Brief or partial loss of consciousness, breathing may be shallow, face pale, skin cold and clammy, pulse may be rapid and weak, nauseous, lack of memory of what happened.
Cramp	Possible dehydration, lack of glucose, electrolyte imbalance, training faults, fatigue, tight clothing particularly socks and shoes, lactic acid build up and cold weather.	Painful, sustained and involuntary contraction. To help ease the pain apply ice first then slowly stretch the muscle involved apply direct pressure over the muscle trigger point and massage using kneading movements. Contraction of the antagonist muscle will also help to relax the cramped muscle.
Dislocation	Part of the capsule surrounding the joint is torn.	Sudden pain, joint gives way, swelling appears. Sometimes can click back into place, especially in the knee.
Exercise-induced asthma	Exercise makes the respiratory system work faster. For some athletes, exercise may cause exercise-induced asthma i.e. asthma that is specifically provoked by the exercise.	Symptoms are wheezing, difficulty in breathing and/or shortness of breath, a constricted sensation in the chest and, sometimes, coughing. Symptoms usually present about 3–8 minutes after beginning the activity.

Injury	Cause	Effects
Fractures	Can be caused as a result of a direct trauma, e.g. impact on the leg or indirect trauma, e.g. an awkward fall.	Compound fracture – ends of bone pierce the skin. Avulsion fractures – bone attached to a muscle or ligament has been torn away.
Hyperventilation	Abnormal loss of carbon dioxide from the blood, leading to chemical changes within the blood	Unnaturally fast breathing, dizziness, trembling and tingling in the hands
Ilio-tibial band syndrome (Runner's knee)	Prolonged running practice and running on cambered roads	Pain after running a certain distance which increases, causing the runner to stop. Pain disappears after rest but recurs if running is resumed. Often occurs when running downhill.
Jogger's nipple	Clothing constantly rubbing against the nipple whilst running.	Very sore nipple area, in acute cases leading to bleeding of the area.
Lateral epicondylitis	Long standing compression found in cycling or from repeated blows in racquet and batting sports.	Pain is felt over the outer elbow area, increasing in intensity on certain movements that stress the tendon. If severe, pain can be felt all around the elbow, resulting in difficulty in writing.
Mallet finger	Rupture in an extensor tendon on the back of a finger caused by e.g. a ball hitting the finger-tip forcing the finger to flex.	Tenderness felt between the nail and the distal joint in the finger and finger tip held slightly flexed when resting.
Periostitis	Inflammation of the periosteum caused by changing from one playing surface to another.	Pain felt on inside of the bone during activity. As activity intensifies pain increases. There is tenderness and swelling.
Ruptured muscles	Burst or tear in the fascia or sheath surrounding a muscle caused by overstretching, overloading, lack of warm up, or weakness due to previous injury or direct impact.	Swelling, bleeding between the ruptured ends of the muscle fibres, could cause restricted joint mobility if rupture occurs at the joint.
Shin splints or Compartment Syndrome	Training too intensely on a hard surface. Common problem with runners.	Pain mainly down lower two-thirds of shin which increases with continued activity; tibialis anterior muscle may be tender and feel swollen.
Sprain	Stretching and tearing of the ligaments within a joint.	Tissue and ligament damage with local swelling and tenderness.

Injury	Cause	Effects
Stitch	Often caused during exercise or after eating a big meal.	Spasms in the diaphragm; usually occur when the athlete is training or working harder than normal or sometimes if they are under tension due to an important race/game etc.
Strain	Tearing or overstretching of muscle fibres.	Pain and swelling causing restricted use.
Stress fractures	Same as shin splints.	Same as shin splints but if no response to treatment after a few sessions, seek medical advice.
Tendinitis	Overuse of a muscle, causing inflammation and scarring of the tendon	Loss of strength in the muscle.
Torn cartilage	Pressure from the bones of the joint when an abnormal force twists the bones against each other abnormally, causing the cartilage tissue to split.	Instant pain, lack of mobility, swelling, stiffness, and weakness in knee.
Torticollis	Violent turning movements of the neck, e.g. when diving or when heading or jumping in football.	Severe pain in the neck and between the nape of the neck and the shoulder. Pain on twisting head to one side.

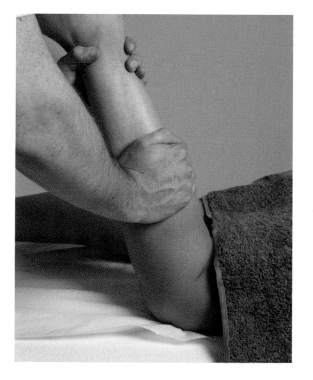

What else should I look for?

Something the client may not be aware of is their posture. At the consultation make sure that you are aware of how they stand and sit. Long-standing postural defects can cause muscle and joint damage. You should also ask about any previous injuries that may have an effect on their body.

Post-treatment procedure

Each individual and each treatment will differ. It would therefore be impossible to suggest a standard post-treatment procedure. However, stretching is always recommended after massage.

HOW EXERCISE AFFECTS THE BODY: SOME SPECIAL CONSIDERATIONS FOR SPORTS MASSAGE

Before treating an athlete or sports person, it helps to understand the effect of exercise and training on different systems of the body. Muscles, for example, need to create energy before that energy can be used in exercise and once the exercise has started by-products from the energy production and muscle use may cause problems such as cramp. Therapists may be treating muscles depleted of energy and overworked. Some muscles will simply be prone to cramp, others will suffer from chronic muscle fatigue. In order to understand how to treat the different muscles worked in exercise it is useful to understand what has happened to them during that exercise session.

How does a muscle move?

Muscles move by contracting. The impulse to contract comes from the nervous system. Motor nerves enter the muscles and split into many nerve endings and each one of these stimulates a single muscle fibre. When the nervous system commands a motor unit (i.e. a motor nerve and all the fibres it supplies) to contract all the muscle fibres of this single motor unit respond together, i.e. 'all-or-nothing'. It is important to remember that the nerve stimulus of one motor unit in the muscle does not mean that the whole muscle is stimulated. For example, at any one time there will be some muscle fibres contracting in all our muscles because this action gives our body normal posture. However, this does not mean that all our muscles are moving – contraction occurs in some muscle fibres even when we think we are still. In order for contraction to cause movement the contracting muscle needs to be attached to a bone (i.e. it is a

skeletal muscle) and pass over a joint. Voluntary muscle (which causes movement and which we control) looks stripey under a microscope. The stripes are made of filaments of proteins called actin and myosin. These proteins run across the muscle fibres in transverse bands. When a muscle contracts the actin filaments slide between the myosin filaments causing a shortening or thickening of the muscle fibres. Fibres shorten when they contract and thus the parts attached to the fibres, such as bones, are pulled in the direction of a contraction and move. Muscles never work in isolation. Any movement is the result of the action of several muscles working together – synergy. Depending on the number of muscle fibres needed for a particular exercise, e.g. weightlifting, the more muscle fibres are required to lift the weight or carry out the exercise, the more motor units are recruited and in some cases the neural discharge frequency is increased (e.g. if more motor units are involved there will be more 'messages' coming from the brain telling them what to do). When effort is sustained, groups of fibres contract in series.

Where does a muscle get energy from?

In order for contraction to take place in a muscle, there must be an adequate supply of blood to provide oxygen and nutrients and to remove the waste products of energy production. Muscles receive their food and oxygen from the arterial capillaries. This is converted into energy by chemical changes. The main chemical substance produced which provides the energy required is a substance called adenosine triphosphate (ATP). If the muscle is well-fed and has plenty of oxygen (e.g. a muscle that has not been overworked recently) its cells will be able to produce ATP quickly and efficiently and therefore have plenty of energy. It will be able to work for longer before getting tired. However, if a muscle is lacking nutrients and oxygen it will not be able to produce ATP efficiently, it will therefore lack energy and the muscle cells will not be able to work for very long before getting tired. Thus a sprinter who has just competed is unlikely to have the energy for another run straightaway because their muscles lack oxygen and nutrients and are less efficient at producing ATP and therefore energy.

Muscle cells can store a small amount of ATP but not very much, so it is important for them to continue producing more ATP in order to keep working. Once ATP is depleted the muscle cells replace it using three different chemical reactions – the aerobic system, anaerobic glycolysis and the creatine phosphate system:

- **aerobic system**

When enough oxygen is transported to a muscle cell for its energy needs there is plenty of ATP and thus plenty of energy. For example, when a muscle is resting plenty of oxygen is being delivered to the cell so the cell has plenty of ATP. Most cells contain mitochondria, also known as the 'power houses' of the cell because aerobic energy production (ATP) takes place in the mitochondria. Cells with lots of mitochondria can produce more aerobic energy.

- **anaerobic system**

When there is not enough energy reaching a muscle cell for its energy needs, for example when a muscle is exercising very hard, the muscle relies on anaerobic and creatine phospate systems to provide ATP. Anaerobic energy is still produced in the cell but not in the mitochondria.

- **creatine phosphate**

Creatine phosphate is a molecule that is used to supply energy when both aerobic and anaerobic systems are exhausted. It is a phosphate and when energy is required it creates energy itself so that it can join up with adenosine diphosphate (ADP) (a molecule containing two phosphates) in order to form adenosine triphosphate (ATP) (a molecule containing three phosphates). It can be broken down very quickly in order to help with ATP production.

So how do muscles get energy during exercise?

- **aerobic system**

When exercise begins after rest, muscle cells will use up their small store of ATP for energy production. As the exercise continues and becomes more intense or vigorous (e.g. speeding up on the treadmill or increasing the weight lifted) the heart and lungs try to speed up the delivery of blood, and therefore oxygen and nutrients, to the mitochondria of the muscles in use so that they can produce the required amount of ATP. This is why your breathing rate and pulse increase during exercise – the body is speeding up the functions which increase oxygen intake and delivery.

- **anaerobic system**

The body will, at some stage, (the time when this happens depends on the exercise carried out, the exerciser's fitness level and the genetic make-up of the person) no longer be able to supply the required amount of oxygen to the muscles in use. This is known as the anaerobic or lactic threshold. This threshold is not reached when the body is working to its maximum level (maximum effort) but before this maximum, usually at around 50-85% of possible maximum effort. At this point the muscle must use the anaerobic system for the production of ATP and energy. The anaerobic system first uses glucose to produce energy. Glucose is a sugar that is stored in the liver in the form of glycogen. When needed it is transported from the liver in the blood to the muscle cells. The muscle then burns the glucose by combining it with oxygen. If the muscles continue to work the anaerobic system will then have to break down creatine phospate in order to produce ATP and thus energy. However, this last stage cannot last for very long because even the muscles of the best-trained athletes can only store enough creatine phospate and ATP for about 10 seconds of exercise at maximal effort.

- **What is maximum effort?**

Maximum effort is measured as follows: it is the amount of weight that one person can lift when all that person's effort goes into that lift i.e. they will not be able to lift it again.

- **Aerobic or anaerobic – which is the most efficient way to produce energy?**

The aerobic system is much more efficient than the anaerobic system. Not only does it produce much more ATP and therefore energy but also its end-products are water and carbon dioxide, neither of which cause muscle fatigue. The by-products of anaerobic ATP production are lactic acid, heat and hydrogen ions. Once the muscle starts to produce lactic acid and other by-products, these products build up in the muscle and prevent the muscle from contracting and functioning properly. However, they cannot be removed until the muscle activity has ceased. Thus, the muscle will soon be unable to contract and the person exercising will feel pain and stiffness. The exerciser will either have to decrease the intensity of the exercise or have a rest.

Finally, when the body is exercising at a rate below the anaerobic (lactic) threshold, i.e. when the body is working at less than 50-85% of maximum effort, ATP is mostly produced by aerobic enzymes which change fat and carbohydrate into energy. However, when the body exercises beyond the anaerobic threshold, ATP is mostly produced by anaerobic enzymes.

How does exercise affect the nervous system?

When the muscles are exercised the nervous system sends impulses to muscles in order to stimulate movement. The hypothalamus in the brain sends a message to the sympathetic nervous system telling it to get the body ready to act. The endocrine system is also stimulated by the hypothalamus to secrete hormones, especially adrenaline. The stimulation of the sympathetic nervous system and the endocrine system has the following effects:

- the cardiovascular system (circulation, respiration and heartbeat) speeds up
- blood is diverted from the skin and internal organs to the muscles so that they have plenty of oxygen for energy production
- the digestive system slows down to prevent wasting energy on food breakdown
- the liver is stimulated to secrete glucose for anaerobic energy production
- the adrenal cortex and medulla are stimulated to secrete hormones, particularly adrenaline which prepares the body for 'fight or flight'
- sweating is stimulated, particularly on the palms of the hands, to help keep the body cool
- salivary glands vasoconstrict (causing a dry mouth feeling)
- pupils of the eyes dilate.

Over-activity of the sympathetic nervous system causes 'nerves' or 'butterflies', a heightened version of the required nervous stimulation which undermines performance. This problem can be controlled by using deep breathing techniques, using the contraction and relaxation of the diaphragm to slow the action of the different systems. In the first instance, this movement of the abdominal muscles pushes up the diaphragm which in turn pushes up on the lungs and the heart, improving their efficiency. Secondly, the pressure on the heart stimulates the vagus nerve which is attached to it. This nerve is part of the parasympathetic nervous system which slows down the movement and actions of the organs of the body. Thus the heart rate slows down and this has a relaxing effect.

How does exercise affect blood pressure?

The cardiovascular system has to work very hard during exercise. It is therefore no surprise that, though exercise is excellent for the heart and lungs, overdoing it can cause certain cardiovascular problems, such as high or low blood pressure.

Blood pressure

Blood pressure is the force that the blood exerts on the vessel walls as it is pumped from the heart. Without the heart blood would not move. Thus blood is always under pressure. There are two 'types' of blood pressure, which are both used in blood pressure measurements: systolic and diastolic. Systolic is the pressure measured when the heart is contracting, i.e. pressure at its highest whereas diastolic is the pressure measured when the heart is relaxing i.e. pressure at its lowest. Normal systolic blood pressure, measured when a person is resting, is about 120/80 i.e. 120 is systolic pressure and 80 is diastolic.

What happens to blood pressure in sport?

Exercise is known to reduce blood pressure overall and is therefore good for anyone suffering from hypertension. However, care should be taken because during the actual exercise the heart rate increases and thus systolic pressure increases. Sometimes the reading may be above 200. This increase is caused by increased heart rate. Diastolic pressure hardly changes during exercise.

THE IMPORTANCE OF DIET AND FLUIDS

Diet

An athlete's diet (meaning what they eat rather than the control of food intake for weight loss) is extremely important to their performance. Without a balanced diet tailored to their particular physical requirements, their body will not be able to perform at optimum efficiency.
NB This section is a brief introduction, not a comprehensive overview of the dietary considerations for an athlete.

The role of carbohydrates

Carbohydrates are the body's energy providers and therefore the most impor-

tant food group for exercise. They are preferable to fat and sugar as they release energy slowly (because they take longer to digest) and therefore they can provide energy over a longer period. Carbohydrates are important because they:

- are the most important energy source for working muscles
- help keep the brain and nervous system working properly
- enable the body to use fat more efficiently.

Carbohydrates are stored in the form of glycogen and this store is the body's most important fuel when exercising. 55-65% of the total calorie intake for any athlete or person exercising should consist of complex carbohydrates such as bread, pasta and cereals which also provide fibre, B vitamins and some trace minerals.

After exercise, carbohydrates are equally important to replace the glycogen that has been used up. Post-exercise is a good time to eat carbohydrates and sugar because the reduced amount of glycogen stimulates the production of glycogen synthase, an enzyme which controls glycogen storage.

What is carbohydrate loading?

Carbohydrate loading is the gradual increase of the amount of carbohydrate consumed in order to increase endurance and therefore performance in certain endurance sports. Over a period of seven days, athletes start eating more and more carbohydrates. This process can boost glycogen stores in muscles by up to 40% – the more glycogen there is in the muscles before exercise, the better the endurance level. Before a competition, usually in the week before an event athletes will start tapering – decreasing their training programmes but increasing their carbohydrate intake.

Which carbohydrates are the best for exercise?

- **Before exercise**: foods which enter the bloodstream slowly and thus provide sustained energy e.g. bananas, pasta, rice (low to moderate glycaemic foods; glycaemic is the rate at which blood glucose rises when a particular carbohydrate food is eaten).
- **During exercise**: energy gels can be eaten because they contain large amounts of sugar which gives instant energy.
- **After exercise**: foods which enter the bloodstream quickly and can

therefore be used to replenish energy levels e.g. high glycaemic index foods such as baked potatoes, cornflakes or honey.

Low glycaemic foods, e.g. pulses, apples, green vegetables, etc. may eliminate the need for consuming carbohydrates during long-term exercise because they maintain normal blood sugar levels.

The role of protein

Eating protein is essential to good health. Proteins are the building material for the body and they are converted into amino acids in order to be used wherever required. Protein is found in dairy products, meat, fish and beans. There are some athletes and training regimes which believe that eating more protein than the body needs will improve performance or health because the extra protein becomes muscle. However, there is no benefit to eating more than is necessary — it has not been proven, for example, that protein supplements, which often contain powdered milk and egg or soya protein can increase muscle growth, strength and endurance — and they could even have a negative effect. Once the body has enough protein, any extra is broken down and eliminated. The part of the protein which contains nitrogen is turned into urea in the liver and is then excreted via the urinary system. This may cause dehydration if insufficient fluids are consumed. The rest of the protein is turned into glucose, a sugar, and used as an energy substitute. This energy may be needed immediately or it may be stored as glycogen. But if the athlete already has a full glycogen store, the body will convert any excess glucose into fat.

The role of fats

Fats are made up of glycerol and fatty acids. There are three different groups of fatty acids - saturated, mono-

sodium. This prevents the stomach from emptying and stops the body from rehydrating. Some athletes think that because they are sweating so much they need to replace the salt but in fact taking these tablets does not have this effect and stops the body getting the fluids it needs.

One way to replace fluids

One way to replace fluids and electrolyte loss is by drinking a dilute sodium/carbohydrate drink (either hypotonic or isotonic) with a sodium concentration of 40-110 mg/100 ml.

You now know what sports massage is, what special considerations are required in treating sportspeople and some of the problems and injuries that affect athletes.

Client Consultation Form – Sports Massage

College Name:
College Number:
Student Name:
Student Number:
Date: Feb

Client Name: Steve
Address: 123 Fit st

Profession:
Tel. No: Day 123456
Eve 123456

PERSONAL DETAILS

Age group: ❏ Under 20   ❏ 20–30   ❏ 30–40   ☑ 40–50   ❏ 50–60   ❏ 60+
Lifestyle: ❏ Active   ❏ Sedentary
Last visit to the doctor: ❏
GP Address:
No. of children (if applicable):
Date of last period (if applicable):

CONTRAINDICATIONS REQUIRING MEDICAL PERMISSION – (select where/if appropriate): Never treat unless the injury has been diagnosed and treatment has been recommended by a medical practitioner.

❏ Pregnancy
❏ Cardio vascular conditions (thrombosis, phlebitis, hypertension, hypotension, heart conditions)
❏ Haemophilia
❏ Any condition already being treated by a GP or another health professional, e.g. Physiotherapist, Osteopath, Chiropractor, Coach
❏ Medical oedema
❏ Osteoporosis
❏ Arthritis
❏ Nervous/Psychotic conditions
❏ Epilepsy
❏ Recent operations
❏ Diabetes
❏ Asthma

❏ Any dysfunction of the nervous system (e.g. Muscular sclerosis, Parkinson's disease, Motor neurone disease)
❏ Bell's Palsy
❏ Trapped/Pinched nerve (e.g. sciatica)
❏ Inflamed nerve
❏ Cancer
❏ Postural deformities
❏ Spastic conditions
❏ Kidney infections
❏ Whiplash
❏ Slipped disc
❏ Undiagnosed pain
❏ When taking prescribed medication
❏ Acute rheumatism

CONTRAINDICTIONS THAT RESTRICT TREATMENT (select where/if appropriate):

❏ Fever
❏ Contagious or infectious diseases
❏ Under the influence of recreational drugs or alcohol
❏ Diarrhoea and vomiting
❏ Skin diseases
❏ Undiagnosed lumps and bumps
❏ Localised swelling
❏ Inflammation
❏ Varicose veins
❏ Pregnancy (abdomen)
❏ Cuts
❏ Bruises
❏ Abrasions

❏ Scar tissues (2 years for major operation and 6 months for a small scar)
❏ Sunburn
❏ Hormonal implants
❏ Abdomen (first few days of menstruation depending how the client feels)
❏ Haematoma
❏ Hernia
❏ Recent fractures (minimum 3 months)
❏ Cervical spondylitis
❏ Gastric ulcers
❏ After a heavy meal

WRITTEN PERMISSION REQUIRED BY:

❏ GP/Specialist   ❏ Informed consent
Either of which should be attached to the consultation form.

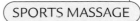

SPORTS MASSAGE

PERSONAL INFORMATION (select if/where appropriate):

Muscular/Skeletal problems: ☐ Back ☑ Aches/Pain ☐ Stiff joints ☐ Headaches

Digestive problems: ☐ Constipation ☐ Bloating ☐ Liver/Gall bladder ☐ Stomach

Circulation: ☐ Heart ☐ Blood pressure ☐ Fluid retention ☐ Tired legs ☐ Varicose veins
☐ Cellulite ☐ Kidney problems ☐ Cold hands and feet ☐ Borderline low blood pressure 110/80

Gynaecological: ☐ Irregular periods ☐ P.M.T ☐ Menopause ☐ H.R.T ☐ Pill ☐ Coil

Other: ....

Nervous system: ☐ Migraine ☐ Tension ☑ Stress ☐ Depression

Immune system: ☐ Prone to infections ☐ Sore throats ☐ Colds ☐ Chest ☐ Sinuses

Regular antibiotic/medication taken? ☐ Yes ☑ No

If yes, which ones: ....

Herbal remedies taken? ☐ Yes ☐ No

If yes, which ones: ....

Ability to relax: ☐ Good ☑ Moderate ☐ Poor

Sleep patterns: ☑ Good ☐ Poor ☐ Average No. of hours 7

Do you see natural daylight in your workplace? ☑ Yes ☐ No

Do you work at a computer? ☑ Yes ☐ No If yes how many hours 1

Do you eat regular meals? ☑ Yes ☑ No

Do you eat in a hurry? ☐ Yes ☑ No

Do you take any food/vitamin supplements? ☑ Yes ☐ No

If yes, which ones: *Multi minerals and vitamins*

How many portions of each of these items does your diet contain per day?

Fresh fruit: *5* Fresh vegetables: *3* Protein: *1* source? *Meat, fish*

Dairy produce: *0* Sweet things: *0* Added salt: *0* Added sugar: *0*

How many units of these drinks do you consume per day?

Tea: *0* Coffee: *0* Fruit juice: *3* Water: *5* Soft drinks: *0* Others: *3*

Do you suffer from food allergies? ☐ Yes ☑ No Bingeing? ☐ Yes ☑ No

Overeating? ☐ Yes ☑ No

Do you smoke? ☑ No ☐ Yes How many per day?

Do you drink alcohol? ☐ No ☑ Yes How many units per day? 2

Do you exercise? ☐ None ☐ Occasional ☐ Irregular ☑ Regular

Types: *Gym, swimming, cycling, tennis, yoga*

What is your skin type? ☑ Dry ☐ Oil ☐ Combination ☐ Sensitive ☐ Dehydrated

Do you suffer/have you suffered from: ☐ Dermatitis ☐ Acne ☐ Eczema ☐ Psoriasis
☐ Allergies ☐ Hay Fever ☐ Asthma ☐ Skin cancer

Stress level: 1–10 (10 being the highest)

At work *6* At home *4*

PHYSICAL EXAMINATION:

Head: normal

Shoulders: normal

Back: slight lordosis

Pelvis: normal

Legs: normal

Feet: slight pronation in left foot

Body alignment/posture: normal

PHYSICAL EXAMINATION

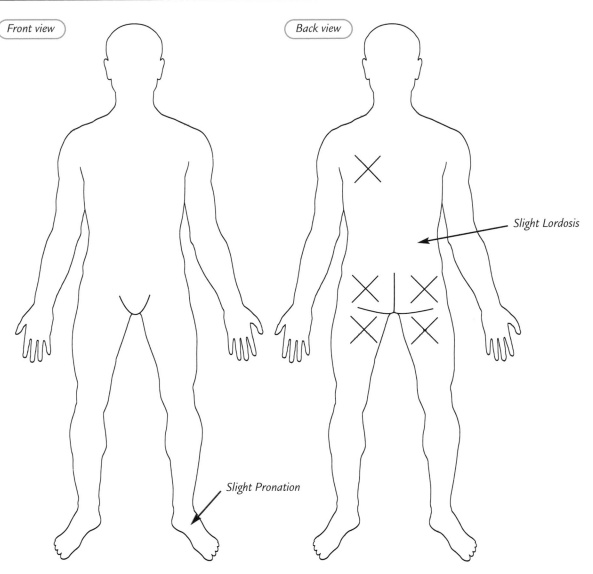

Front view

Back view

Slight Lordosis

Slight Pronation

Assessment: After completing the consultation form, in which I found out that Steve was a keen athlete and had no major health problems, I asked him to strip down to his underpants and to put the towel round his waist ready for me to assess his posture and problem areas.
I asked Steve to stand relaxed allowing me to make a visual observation of his body alignment before making a more detailed analysis with my hands. Steve has good muscle definition all over and has a slight curvature of the spine in the lumbar region. Apart from that, his posture is good.

He was then asked to lie down on the couch face down, placing a rolled up towel under his shoulders and ankles for relaxation. Skin rolling technique was used to see if there were any areas of thickened fascia and poor elasticity as this could restrict movement. The fascia around the lumbar region and up most of the thoracic region had poor mobility. More mobility was felt near the top thoracic and the base of the neck. On palpating the area, tension nodules were felt in the lower trapezius muscle around T4 – T7. No other discrepancies were found.

On his legs thickened fascia could be felt at the top of both legs and around the buttock area, particularly the left buttock. Tightness in the muscles was felt in the upper hamstrings and gluteals on palpation

Rationale for Treatment: As the lower back felt tight with some thickened fascia I have decided to use some Connective Tissue Massage (CTM) around this area to relieve the congestion and tension. The CTM will be performed using fingers, hands and lower arm at the appropriate places. Circular frictions will also be used to release any tension areas in the muscles.

For the upper back, as well as using CTM, I will apply some Soft Tissue Release (STR) to help release the tension found around the lower trapezius muscle helping to loosen up the scapula.

For his hamstrings and gluteals I am going to use Neuromuscular Technique (NMT) to try to reduce the tension in the area, some cross frictions if necessary and strain counter strain (STS).

Throughout the massage I will go back to the skin rolling technique to check the fascia tissue is responding.

Treatment: I told Steve that throughout the treatment I will be asking him about the pain/discomfort he felt and at what level he finds it from 1-10, 10 being the most painful.

Using the skin rolling technique starting from the right side, I gradually worked my way in towards the spine noticing the nearer I got to the spine the tighter the skin was, meaning the fascia tissue was tight. Steve stated that at the point just before the lumbar spine the pain was up to about 7 with a slight burning sensation felt. I used the effleurage movement over the whole area to relax it.

This time I went over the same area rolling with my fingers at an angle of about 30o which appeared to release the tension considerably and far less pain was felt. The left side was then massaged using the same techniques paying close attention to the tight areas. By using the different parts of my fingers, hands and forearm the muscles appeared to respond quite quickly and much more movement was felt at the end of the 15 minutes spent on the lower back. Moving up to the thoracic, the left side again felt tight so I initially palpated the area using the pads of my fingers. Then by applying CTM with the heel of my hand and circular movements with my forearm, particularly around the lower scapula, the tension nodules were soon released. STR was then used on the scapula to loosen the surrounding muscles achieved by raising Steve's left arm therefore shortening the muscles, using the heel of my left arm to lock and glide over the muscles to lengthen them. The right side was then treated in the same way with much less tension felt and much less work needed to release the fascia.

For the legs and gluteals, again skin rolling was used moving up the thighs and over the buttocks. The skin appeared tight in both hamstrings and gluteals, Steve commenting that the left side felt much more painful. I then palpated the area on the right thigh moving up from just above the popliteal space, up the biceps femoris muscle and into the buttock area using the pads of my thumbs. NMT was then applied using the pads of my thumbs again gradually increasing the pressure for 60 seconds the first time with little increase but the second time increasing the pressure and holding for 90 seconds. Steve found the second time the pain had faded considerably. The treatment was repeated on the left thigh and buttock, but this time Steve commented that the pain, although had faded, was still quite intense so cross-fibre frictions were used to try to loosen and free the adhesions in the area.

I finished off with strain counter strain (SCS) which Steve commented really felt good and he could feel the difference in his thighs. He could feel he was more flexible.

How the client felt during the treatment: Steve did feel pain and burning sensations a few times during the treatment particularly during CTM. This was probably due to me having to apply some more pressure to some areas to release the excess tension. However, he did say he could feel the tension going from the tense areas during the treatment.

How the client felt after the treatment: Steve feels relief from the tightness in his lower back, thighs and buttocks, particularly on the left side feeling much more flexible, despite the pain, he has enjoyed the experience.

Home care advice given: As Steve does not drink much water I have advised him to increase this to at least 2 litres and while he is exercising to keep drinking water to ensure he keeps hydrated. Because Steve has tight back muscles I have advised him to stretch out his back every morning and evening and whenever he feels it tightening up.

For his lower back he should:

1) Kneel on all fours, inhale contract the abdominals and round the back. Hold for about 5 seconds then relax the abdominals returning back to a flat back. Repeat this movement at least 10 times morning and night.

2) Stand with feet hip distance apart, put hands above your head, left hand gripping right wrist, pull right hand over to the left side as far as you can. This will stretch the side of the body and the latissimus dorsi. Repeat 10 times both sides.

If he feels his back tightening up at work he can:

1) Sit on a chair with legs slightly apart, exhale, extend the torso, bend at the hips and lower the stomach between the thighs. Hold for 10 seconds, repeat 10 times.

2) Sit on a straight backed chair, turn to the right, place hands on the back of the chair, exhale keeping feet flat on the floor and buttocks on seat. Push right hip forward and press right elbow into the body.

And for his thighs and buttocks I suggested after a hot bath or shower

1) Sit on the floor, one leg straight the other bent at the knee with the heel touching the inner leg. Keeping the outside of the thigh and calf of the bent leg on the floor reach up, inhale, then as you lower the upper torso breath out and try to put your chin on your knee. Hold for 30 seconds.

2) Lie on the floor, legs extended, flex one knee, raise it to your chest and grasp with opposite hand. Exhale and pull your knee across your body to the floor keeping elbows, head and shoulders flat on the floor.

I also advised Steve to swim at least twice during the week as this would help with any potential stiffness reoccurring.

Reflective practice: I was very pleased with this session and could feel I'd managed to release much of the tension Steve had when he arrived. When Steve rotated his hips he said his lower back felt much freer, although he could still feel the stiffness in his thighs and buttocks on the left side, but the right felt much better.

Although Steve did not have a specific injury the tightness in his lower back, buttocks and thighs was preventing him from carrying out his normal exercising to a certain extent. He now feels he has more mobility.

I have advised him that he might feel some pain tomorrow as I have worked quite deeply into his muscles and generally an aching feeling is felt for about 24 hours after treatment. I have arranged to see Steve again in 5 days' time to make sure he is not stiffening up again and to help prevent the stiffness reoccurring.

SPORTS MASSAGE FOLLOW-UP SHEET 1

Assessment: Steve was walking noticeably more freely when he came into the room which meant his back, buttocks and thighs were not as tight. He also got onto the couch and settled without as much difficulty appearing more mobile and less restricted in his movements. Steve said there was a huge improvement in his back, not feeling stiff in the mornings, but his thighs were still causing him a few problems with mobility. He has found the exercises I gave him very useful particularly doing them in the mornings for his back, but hasn't been too keen on doing anything after his evening shower. He has been working long hours since his last appointment and has found that sitting in his seat at work, his back has started to tighten up and his legs and buttocks felt like they were seizing up on him. Because of his work commitments he hasn't been swimming as I suggested. Standing on the right side I palpated the area checking for any signs of tension, no nodules were discovered. Skin rolling in the lower back, tightness was felt with the back feeling much tighter the further up the back I went. Between the spine and the scapula the tissue felt fibrous and thick with the skin not moving smoothly. Steve felt as if I was pinching him which gave him some discomfort. Steve works at a computer most of the day and doesn't feel his posture is good so this could be the reason why his upper back is tight along with the base of his neck.

On his thighs again skin rolling was carried out and again tightness in the deeper muscles was felt particularly in the left thigh and buttock.

Rationale for Treatment: I am going to apply CTM to the whole back, light circular friction movements to the areas of tension to help loosen and stimulate the muscles and STR around the scapula. For the buttocks and thighs I am going to apply NMT but this time include Muscle Energy Technique (MET) to help separate the muscle fibres and remove adhesions and fibrous tissue.

Treatment: With Steve lying on his stomach and me on his left side I started to warm the tissues in his back using double handed effleurage starting lightly but gradually getting deeper to improve circulation and to ensure no discomfort was felt.

I then used my right lower arm, starting at the lower back and moving up the back, meeting resistance in the thoracic area. This was repeated 3 more times until the resistance had reduced. I gently effleuraged the area then moved across the whole of the lower back, varying my pressure and movements until the skin became more mobile and resistance was no longer felt. Where there had been excess tension present redness had appeared due to the increase in blood flow.

Moving up the spine using light circular friction thumb movements I felt tension, so changed to using my forearm moving up the groove of the back releasing the tension. Resistance was felt towards the upper part of the thoracic vertebrae so changed the angle and applied deeper pressure and circular frictions for about 10 seconds. This was repeated twice more before moving to the top of the table and approaching the area from a different direction. CTM was applied to the area between the scapulae on both sides, effleuraged to drain away the toxins and then rolling to reassess the tissue. Light STR was then applied to the shoulder area on both sides one after the other with Steve's arm raised to shorten the muscles, locked down with the heel of my hand and then my hand moved slowly along the muscle fibres as the arm was being lowered.

For his thighs I also started to warm the tissues using double handed effleurage starting lightly but gradually getting deeper to improve circulation and to ensure no discomfort was felt. Using my right forearm I moved up the thigh and buttocks which Steve found particularly painful at the top of his left thigh. I decided to do CTM again on his thighs and buttocks as this would help to stretch the muscle fibres and release any tension within. I also included MET on his thighs to help lengthen the muscles. This was followed with petrissage all over and then light hacking and cupping to bring the blood to the surface. I then did skin rolling to check the tension was subsiding - much more movement was felt in the tissues - finishing with effleurage helping to remove the toxins. Steve has very red areas around his upper back due to the amount of work I have done in that area releasing the tension. The tension in the back, buttocks and thighs has improved as can be seen by the skin rolling where the tissue has moved much more easily.

How the client felt during the treatment: Steve felt at some points in his upper back and buttocks slight pain

and pinching but overall it was not as uncomfortable as the last session. He really liked the thumb circles up either side of the spine and the MET on his thighs as he felt he was contributing to the massage and to his body helping himself to improve.

How the client felt after the treatment: Steve felt relief from the aching in his upper back particularly around the shoulders and felt much more relaxed. He felt his thighs were much looser and when walking around felt he could swing his legs much more easily.

Home care advice given: I advised Steve to continue the exercises I gave him last time as this will help with his flexibility and release initial tension from the back. Another suggestion to ease the tension across the shoulder blades would be to grip a door frame and then lean back stretching the teres minor and infraspinatus muscles. This along with the other exercises should be done at least 10 times morning and evening to get the most benefit out of them.

For his buttocks and thighs I suggested he swing his legs back and forth about 50 times each leg which would help to loosen the muscles particularly in the mornings when the stiffness is always at its worst.

Reflective practice: This session again went well and I feel I achieved what I set out to do. Steve is very happy with the results, feeling more relaxed and less stiff. The CTM seems to work very well and Steve responds really quickly with only having to apply a little more pressure to reach beyond the superficial layers. Steve has booked in for another treatment in 5 days time

SPORTS MASSAGE FOLLOW-UP SHEET 2

Assessment: Steve is feeling much better, just feeling some tightness in his upper back and his buttocks after sitting down for too long. He has been for a swim twice since his last visit and feels it has really helped keep the tension at bay. Once Steve was comfortable on the couch in prone position, I started to palpate the back using the pads of my fingers. There were no signs of heat in the lower back but still some signs of tightness, also around the base of the neck and in his buttocks particularly the left side still; the thighs felt much more relaxed and normal. Nodules were still present around the medial border of the right scapula. Skin rolling all the way up the back and down the buttocks and thighs helping to assess the mobility of the tissue which was much improved compared to the first session. Most of the problems appear to be around the base of Steve's neck and his left buttock.

Rationale for Treatment: CTM, light friction and STR will be applied on the back to give a deep massage. Circular friction movements will be used around the medial border of the right scapula. I will also apply pertrissage and tapotement movements to improve circulation, stimulate blood flow and help loosen up any tight muscles remaining. For his buttocks and thighs I will apply STR and NMT along with some petrissage, percussion and effleurage

Treatment: After using effleurage on the back I used petrissage movements up the sides and across the shoulders increasing pressure where needed. Hacking and cupping were applied on the sides of the back and finished off with effleurage. CTM was applied with my forearm around the lower back moving up towards the neck. I got Steve to bring his right arm behind his back, I rested his elbow on my knee helping to lift the scapula and used circular thumb friction movements along the medial border. On releasing Steve's arm I effleuraged the area draining any excess toxins away from the area and tested for any remaining nodules present. None were found. CTM was applied to the upper back using the heel of my hand for deeper pressure, petrissage to the tops of the shoulders and completing the massage with effleurage over the whole area.

For his buttocks and thighs I used effleurage to warm the area, some petrissage and then NMT. I had to apply deep pressure to get to the deeper fibres to release them and held the pressure for 90 seconds. The tension in Steve's muscles responded well, so only light cross fibre frictions were applied. I then decided to include MET again as Steve really enjoyed it and it was a good way of assessing if his muscles were responding as I thought. I finished again with petrissage, hacking, cupping and effleurage

On reassessing the whole area using skin rolling, all areas feel more mobile, tension nodules appear to have disappeared and Steve's flexibility has improved.

How the client felt during the treatment: Steve really enjoyed the massage, feeling no discomfort, enjoying the movements around his neck and upper back. His neck and shoulders felt much looser, his buttocks did not feel as tight and his thighs felt normal again.

How the client felt after the treatment: Steve really enjoyed the massage, the pressure felt good and he felt really relaxed and happy.

Home care advice given: I told Steve to continue with his exercises and to try and swim at least twice a week to release any possible tension that could be building up. He must drink at least 2 litres of water to keep hydrated and ensure he always has a bottle of water when doing any exercise. I have advised him to try to stand up and walk around rolling his shoulders and arms at least every 30 minutes if he is sitting in front of his desk on the computer to release any tension that could be building up. I have also advised him to have a regular massage, at least once a month, to ensure that any nodules are dispersed quickly before getting too established.

Reflective practice: Steve feels much more relaxed with no tension nodules felt in his back, buttocks or thighs. I felt this session was very rewarding with being able to release all the tension found easily using the techniques explained.

Overall conclusion: The movements used during these sessions have been very successful. The various methods of applying CTM were very good in releasing the tightness quickly, following up with the STR. The SCS, NMT and MET were all very encouraging in solving Steve's problems. The exercises given for home care were adhered to by Steve which was a great help for recovery and if he continues doing them will help prevent any problems for quite some time.

DON'T FORGET NOW YOU CAN USE A RANGE OF ONLINE LEARNING RESOURCES FOR JUST £10 (NORMAL RRP £20)

50% OFF! FULL ACCESS

The Massage e-Learning Resource has been designed to enhance your learning experience

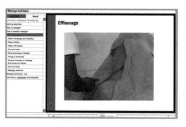

☐ Bring knowledge to life with videos of each technique as well as a full massage routine

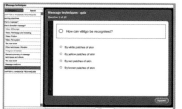

☐ Manage your learning with step-by-step modules and integrated 'classroom' sessions

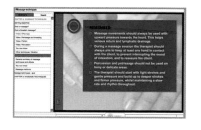

☐ Absorb information on key topics with interactive exercises and learning activities

To login to use these **e-learning resources**, visit **www.emspublishing.co.uk/massage** and follow the onscreen instructions

AN INTRODUCTORY GUIDE TO

Massage

12 Other complementary therapies

In Brief

Massage is only one of many complementary and holistic therapies. This chapter gives a brief overview of others. Some massage therapists combine therapies in treatment. For example aromatherapy and acupressure which are both compatible with massage treatments.

Learning objectives

The target knowledge of this chapter is:
● the definition of other complementary therapies.

AROMATHERAPY

Aromatherapy massage uses the pharmacological, physical and aromatic effects of essential oils for relaxation and the improvement of physical and emotional well-being. Using a blend of carrier and essential oils in the correct dilutions, the aromatherapist massages an affected area or the whole body depending on the client's requirements.

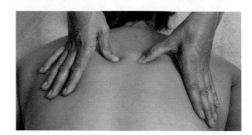

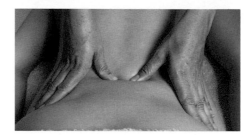

How does aromatherapy massage work?

Aromatherapy massage uses some of the classic Swedish massage techniques to aid relaxation, improve circulation and lymphatic drainage, improve suppleness and aid the release of muscular tension. It combines this with a particular massage medium, a blend of essential oils and carrier oil, to affect the body physically, pharmacologically and psychologically. The warmth of the therapist's hands helps to move the oil across the skin, enabling absorption through the skin and inhalation through the nose. Once the massage oil has been absorbed into the body, the essential oils affect the body in different ways depending on which ones have been used.

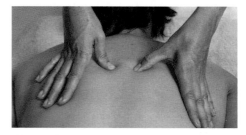

What is an essential oil?

An essential oil is an aromatic, volatile substance that is extracted from plant material. It comes from various parts of the plant, such as the flowers, leaves or bark and some plants produce more than one essential oil. These are similar to animal hormones and are sometimes referred to as the plant's life force. Essential oils have tiny molecules and are thus easily absorbed. It is important to use good quality essential oils because their therapeutic benefits derive from their origins and chemical make-up. Adulterated oils (oils that have been

changed in some way) and synthetic copies will not have the same effects.

What does it do?

An essential oil has three effects on the body – pharmacological, physiological and psychological.

- **Pharmacological**

Essential oils are chemical substances and so are humans. Once an essential oil is absorbed into the body, its chemicals enter the bloodstream, and are circulated around the rest of the body, where they interact with our own chemistry. For example, the nervous system relies on messages from all over the body, delivered by neurotransmitters along the length of our nerves. These neurotransmitters are chemicals and their messages will be subtly altered by the presence of an essential oil.

- **Physiological**

The way our body works is known as its physiology. Essential oils have an effect on this because they interact with the chemical messages and impulses that our body uses to work. An essential oil with sedative properties will thus send a sedating message around the body, soothing nerves and helping relaxation.

- **Psychological**

As well as being absorbed by the skin the essential oil is inhaled through the nose and into the olfactory tract. The heat of the massage releases the oil's molecules into the air and the nose inhales them. These molecules travel up the nose to the olfactory membranes which connect to the olfactory nerves. Once the molecules have been registered by the membranes and then the nerves, a message travels to the brain. The information is received by the limbic area of the brain, the area associated with memory, emotions and instincts. Smell is thus closely linked to emotions. Depending on the oil and how it is interpreted (e.g. a nice smell, a horrible smell, one associated with a happy holiday) the brain sends different responses around the body. It is thus very important to ensure that the oils used in a massage are chosen in consultation with the client – a massage with a scent that a client dislikes will not be relaxing!

If they are chemicals, are they safe?

Used properly, essential oils are very safe because they are diluted and only applied in tiny amounts. However, they are extremely concentrated and potentially toxic and should therefore only be used diluted and not applied directly to the skin or taken internally. The following essential oils are not recommended for use under any circumstances:

Aniseed	Arnica
Bitter almond	Bitter fennel
Camphor	Cassia
Cinnamon bark	Dwarf pine
Elecampane	Horseradish
Hyssop	Mustard
Origanum	Pennyroyal
Rue	Sage
Sassafras	Savin
Savory (winter and summer)	
Southernwood	Tansy
Thuja	Wintergreen
Wormseed	Wormwood

You now know what an essential oil is and how it affects the body. The next section explains how to blend oils and the techniques used in aromatherapy massage.

What is a carrier oil?

A carrier oil is a base oil which is blended with essential oils to create a massage medium. Carrier oils are usually of plant, vegetable or nut origin and need to be either neutral or without a strong scent so that they do not interfere with the effect of the essential oil. Recommended carrier oils include grapeseed, sweet almond, sunflower and peach kernel. Mineral oils such as baby oil are not recommended for use.

Why use a carrier oil?

Essential oils are concentrated and therefore expensive. It is dangerous to use them undiluted on the skin because they are so strong and potentially toxic. Finally, the word oil in the name is a bit of a misnomer: an essential oil is really the essence of a plant, a non-greasy, volatile substance which would not go very far in a massage. The carrier oil literally carries the essence and spreads it all over the body in a safely diluted and affordable form. The carrier oil has large molecules and is therefore not so easily absorbed by the skin.

How much of each type of oil should be used in a blend?

The essential oil should be blended with the chosen carrier oil in the following dilutions:

- 2 drops of essential oil to 5ml (1 teaspoon) carrier oil for adults
- 1 drop of essential oil to 5ml (1 teaspoon) carrier oil for the elderly/frail, babies or children
- 6 drops of essential oil to 15ml (three teaspoons or 1 tablespoon) carrier oil
- 1ml of essential oil to 50ml (10 teaspoons) carrier oil.

No more than eight drops of essential oil should be used per treatment.

Once blended, essential oils will share the shelf life of the carrier oil they are mixed with, but as they are volatile it is best not to mix more than is needed. The following suggested amounts will obviously need to be adapted for smaller/larger frames, children and the elderly:

- a face massage requires 5ml carrier oil (and only 1 drop essential oil)
- a full body massage requires 20-30 ml carrier oil
- a specific area of the body (e.g. hands, feet, arm, neck) may require from 5-15 ml oil.

Which techniques are used in aromatherapy massage?

Since relaxation is the main goal of aromatherapy massage, the main techniques used are effleurage, petrissage, lymph drainage and acupressure.

When is aromatherapy massage not recommended?

As with other massage types there are times when aromatherapy massage is not recommended. The main contra-indications are listed in Chapter 5. However, with aromatherapy massage particular care should be taken when treating clients who are allergic, atopic, epileptic or pregnant. Pregnancy is contraindicated in the first trimester and from then on mandarin is the only oil recommended for use.

OTHER COMPLEMENTARY THERAPIES

Acupuncture

An ancient Chinese therapy, now being used more and more in the West, acupuncture is the insertion of very fine needles into the skin at certain points to help relieve pain and improve the body's own healing mechanisms. The points are on meridians (energy channels). If there is a blockage in energy then a part of the body connected to that meridian may become ill or weak. The needles are thought to release the blockage and help the body to heal itself.

Acupressure

A manual pressure technique using the hands, elbows, arms, knees and feet to stimulate and rebalance body energy.

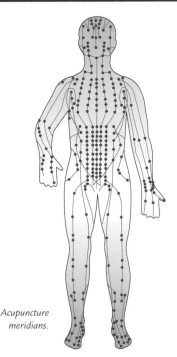

Acupuncture meridians.

Working in the same way as Shiatsu, acupressure clears blockages in key body points allowing energy to flow freely along the meridians.

Alexander technique

The Alexander technique encourages healing and better health through better posture and awareness of how the body is used. It is especially useful for backache and headaches. It was developed by an actor called Frederick Mathias Alexander who discovered that improving his posture stopped him losing his voice.

Ayurvedic medicine

Ayurveda means knowledge (ayur) of life (veda). Body harmony and good health are achieved through proper diet, exercise, lifestyle and meditation, specific to a client's constitution or mix of doshas, or body elements – vata,pitta and kapha. It focuses on rebalance or attunement to the correct dosha rather than the exclusive treatment of symptoms. Widely practised in India, it is a philosophy and a lifestyle as well as a medicine.

Bach flower remedies

Dr Edward Bach, a doctor and a practising homeopath, turned away from both traditional medicine and homeopathy believing that there was a more natural and holistic way to treat illness. He developed 38 remedies, which are infusions of plants with water and alcohol, based on his research in the countryside. The remedies aim to treat mental and emotional problems, which often precede and cause physical symptoms.

Bodywork

There are various forms of bodywork, many with cultural foundations such as Shiatsu, Lomi Lomi, Kahuna massage, Amma massage, Marma Point massage, Heller work, Rolfing and holistic massage. While these types focus on treatment of the body through manipulation of the soft tissues others, such as chiropractic and osteopathy, focus on manipulation of the joints.

Bowen technique

The Bowen technique, developed in Australia by Thomas A. Bowen, aims to rebalance the body holistically using gentle moves on tissues. A Bowen practitioner can feel whether muscles are stressed or tense and use the moves to release this build-up. The light rolling movements stimulate the body's energy flows. It is not a massage or a manipulation but a gentle process that encourages the body to heal itself.

Colour therapy

Colour therapy is the therapeutic use of colour and light applied to specific points (acupoints) to rebalance body energy. Performed using coloured fabrics, candles, liquids, and gemstones often in the shape of wands or prisms. Also used as part of Ayurvedic medicine; the seven main chakras have specific colours associated with them.

Chiropractic

A chiropractor manipulates the joints of the body, specifically the spine, in order to relieve pain. It works on the basis that pain is often caused by a nerve which is not functioning properly and thus the spine, which the central nervous system runs through, is the focus of the therapy. It is especially useful for any lower back and neck pains as well as headaches.

Crystal Therapy

A vibrational therapy involving placement of specific crystals on the chakras to rebalance the body energies and improve health. Crystals such as

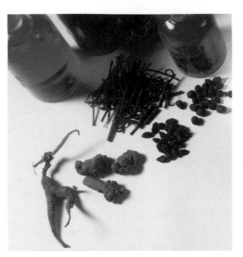

Some herbs used in Chinese medicine.

rose quartz and amethyst are used during treatments.

Ear Candling
Also known as thermo-auricular therapy, ear candling involves placing a specialised candle in the ear canal and lighting the opposite end. This is thought to create a low-level vacuum that draws out earwax and impurities, relieving pressure in the head and sinuses.

Herbalism
Herbalism is the use of plants, usually the whole plant, to make herbal remedies. It is an ancient, traditional medicine — what is now considered traditional medicine only replaced it in the last three hundred years.

Homeopathy
Homeopathy treats like with like. By using minute doses of the bacteria, virus or substance which has caused the problem in the first place (i.e. cat hair in a remedy for an allergy to cat hairs), the treatment builds up the patient's resistance and immunity to the problem substance or bacteria. Many homeopathic remedies have to be used and even stored well away from strong smells because such smells can reduce their effectiveness.

Hypnotherapy
A treatment where the therapist induces a deep state of relaxation in the client by using a soothing, monotonous tone of voice. Thought to bring about a different level of consciousness where the client becomes receptive to suggestion. Commonly used to assist with changing habits such as smoking or overeating and states such as anxiety.

Iridology
By studying the irises (the coloured parts of the eyes) of a patient and noting any changes, iridologists can diagnose physical and psychological problems.

Kinesiology
Kinesiology is a holistic treatment that focuses on testing the muscles and energy meridians to discover and then treat the body's imbalances on all levels: chemically, energetically, physically and mentally. Using different positions and the application of pressure to the limbs, the kinesiologist can determine whether there are any energy blocks in the body and correct them through firm massage. Kinesiology is preventative and, like many complementary therapies, aims to treat the whole person.

Naturopathy
Naturopathy is a therapy that combines 'natural' healing practices such as herbal remedies, hydrotherapy and diet with modern methods of testing, such as x-rays to ascertain problems and rebalance health.

Neurolinguistic Programming
Developed in the 1970s by Richard Bandler and John Grinder, NLP focuses on changing pattens of metal and emotional behaviour through self-awareness and effective communication. Thought to be useful for the treatment of

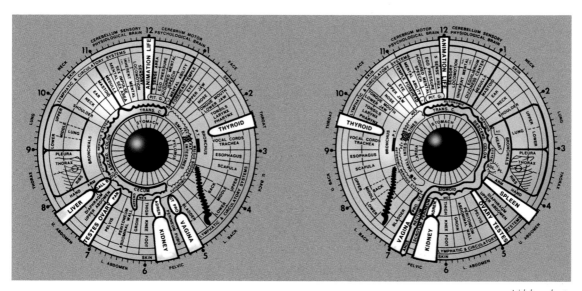

Iridology charts.

nervous system disorders such as phobia and depression.

Osteopathy

Like a chiropractor, an osteopath manipulates the joints of the body. Osteopaths work on the basis that the body's structure and function are interdependent: if the structure is damaged in any way it will affect the function. By manipulating joints and bones they can correct structural problems which will improve the body's function.

Physiotherapy

Physiotherapy uses physical exercises, massage and the application of pressure to relieve physical pain and muscular tension. It is often used to re-educate the body in cases of major surgery, illness, or an accident.

Reflexology

This holistic therapy treats the whole person, particularly weak or ill areas, by using the feet as 'maps' of the body. On the feet there are points or zones which correspond to organs and systems of the body. By pressing on one of these points, the corresponding organ in the body is affected. For example, pressing on the tip of the big toe will cause a response in the brain and, vice versa, if there is a problem with the brain the reflexologist will recognise the symptoms of this in the big toe. This relationship, between a point on the foot and another part of the body is known as a reflex. A trained reflexologist uses finger or thumb pressure on each of the zones to find the problem areas. He or she then applies more pressure which helps the corresponding part of the body to heal. Some professionals use reflexology techniques during massage treatment.

Reiki/spiritual healing

Reiki means universal life force energy in Japanese and Reiki healers act as channels for this universal energy to pass into the patient/client. By using hands in certain positions on different parts of the body, the healer is said to draw energy to the body, promoting healing, balance and relaxation.

Shiatsu

Shiatsu is a form of acupressure: the use of finger or thumb pressure on points along meridians (energy channels) to help relieve pain and encourage the body to heal itself. The pressure points are the same as those used in acupuncture.

OTHER COMPLEMENTARY THERAPIES

Stone Therapy

The use of heated and cooled stones applied through massage or indirect application to the body to relax and rejuvenate muscles and circulation. Different temperatures stimulate the body's natural healing responses to balance mind, body and spirit. Also known as geothermal therapy.

Subtle energy/vibrational medicine

A form of therapy that views the body as an 'energy system'. It uses natural resonance to restore the flow of body energy; therapies such as acupuncture, aromatherapy, Bach flower therapy, chakra rebalancing, channeling, colour therapy, crystal healing, absent healing, flower essence therapy, homeopathy, reiki or polarity therapy harness subtle energy frequencies and channel them to induce healing.

Thai Massage

The traditional healing massage of Thailand (commonly known as Thai massage) originated in India during the Buddha's lifetime, over 2500 years ago. As Buddhism spread from India, so did this form of healing massage. Monks in Thailand originally used this therapy as one element of their healing practices, which consisted of dietary advice, the use of herbs, meditation, and what we now call Thai massage. This form of massage involves manipulation using stretching techniques and gentle pressure along the meridians or energy lines of the body. (See Ayurvedic Medicine.)

Therapeutic touch

A therapy that involves gentle 'laying-on' of hands to invoke a healing response. The therapist uses their hands to detect imbalances in the body.

*Yoga posture —
a shoulder stand.*

Traditional Chinese Medicine

TCM is an ancient system of health care from China that is based on a concept of balanced qi or vital energy, which is believed to flow throughout the body. The opposing forces of yin (negative energy) and yang (positive energy) influence qi, and these forces are thought to regulate the balance of mind, body and spirit. A disruption in qi brings about disease. TCM practitioners use herbal and nutritional therapy, exercise, meditation, acupuncture, and massage to restore balance and health.

Vertical Reflexology

This therapy focuses on the weight bearing dorsal reflexes rather than the soles of the feet. Treatments are performed with the client standing to access deep reflexes. The feet are thought to be more sensitive as a result of weight bearing, and treatments are normally shorter in duration than classical reflexology.

Yoga/meditation

Both yoga and meditation have long been known to have beneficial, holistic effects and they are very useful self-help therapies. They teach the learner to have control of the body and mind. Yoga does this through physical exercise, including adopting different postures, relaxation techniques and breathing exercises. Meditation uses different focuses (such as visualisation, a candle, a mantra) to help a person find calm and a sense of their own centre. Meditation has the physiological effects of a short sleep, i.e. the body goes into the healing and recharging mode it adopts when we sleep, allowing the muscles to relax and the circulation to become more efficient.

You now know details about several other complementary therapies.

THE LIBRARY
TOWER HAMLETS COLLEGE
POPLAR HIGH STREET
LONDON E14 0AF
Tel: 0207 510 7763

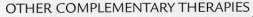
OTHER COMPLEMENTARY THERAPIES

Bibliography

- Beck, Mark, *The Theory and Practice of Therapeutic Massage*, Tarrytown, NY: Milady, 1988.
- Maxwell-Hudson, Claire, *The Complete Book of Massage*, London: Dorling Kindersley, 1988.
- McGuinness, Helen, *Holistic Therapies*, London: Hodder and Stoughton, 2000.
- McGuinness, Helen, *Indian Head Massage: Therapy Basics*, London: Hodder and Stoughton, 2000.
- Mitchell, Stewart, *Massage: a Practical Introduction*, Shaftesbury: Element, 1992.
- Tucker, Louise, *An Introductory Guide to Anatomy and Physiology*, London: EMS Publishing, 2012.
- Tucker, Louise, *An Introductory Guide to Aromatherapy*, London: EMS Publishing, 2012.
- Wittlinger, H. and G., *Introduction to Dr. Vodder's Manual Lymph Drainage, Vol. 1: Basic Course*, Heildelberg: Haug, 1985

Glossary

Active movement: movement which requires client's participation

Acupressure : ancient Chinese therapy using thumb or finger pressure at acupoints along energy meridians in the body to unblock energy

Acupuncture: ancient Chinese therapy using needles inserted at acupoints along energy meridians in the body to unblock energy

Adenosine Triphosphate (ATP): a high energy phosphate molecule required to provide energy for cellular function

After care advice: advice given after a treatment to help maintain the effects of the treatment and the possible reactions that could occur

Allopathic: traditional Western medicine

Alexander technique: encourages healing and better health through improved posture and awareness of how the body is used

Amma: Ancient Chinese massage relying on treating specific points on the body

Aromatherapy: the use of essential oils for relaxation and the improvement of physical and emotional well-being

Ayurvedic medicine: The Ayurveda (from Sanskrit, *ayur* meaning 'life' and *veda* 'knowledge') is an ancient medical text about the arts of healing and prolonging life and it still forms the basis of much medical knowledge in India today.

Bach flower remedies: an infusion of plants with water and alcohol to treat mental and emotional problems

Blood pressure: the force that the blood exerts on the walls of the blood vessels as transmitted from the heart

Bowen technique: rebalancing the body holistically using gentle moves on tissues

Carbohydrates: are the body's energy providers

Carrier oil: neutral vegetable oil used in a blend with essential oil as a massage medium

Cellulite: a type of fat, mainly affecting women, causing dimpling and puckering of the skin. The formation of cellulite is linked to the hormones oestrogen and progesterone

Champissage: a percussion massage movement using both hands together in a 'prayer' position in a rhythmic movement

Chiropractic: manipulating the joints of the body, especially the spine, to relieve pain

Compression: the application of pressure to the body using the heel of the hand or fist to push the muscle tissue against the bone

Connective Tissue Massage (CTM): a form of stretching to release the fluids trapped within the connective tissue between the muscle fibres

Consultation: discussion with client to find out their needs and requirements and to find out any contraindications

Contraindication: reason why treatment cannot take place

Deep: below the surface; area furthest from skin

Desquamation: Natural shedding of skin cells

Effleurage: a gentle, relaxing stroke generally used at the beginning and end of a massage sequence or work on one particular section

Essential fatty acids: fats that cannot be produced by the body so must be supplied by the diet. These are Omega 3 and Omega 6

Essential oil: an aromatic, volatile substance extracted from plant material, with tiny molecules making it easy to be absorbed by the skin

Fats: an essential nutrient that provides energy, energy storage, and insulation and contour to the body

Friction: firm, rubbing technique which pushes layers of tissue against each other in order to stretch muscle fibres and release tension. Used as focus on specific area of body.

Galen: Greek who worked for the Roman Emperor, wrote many medical books stressing the use of massage for health purposes.

Herbalism: the use of plants to make herbal remedies

Herodicus: fifth-century physician and teacher of Hippocrates, wrote about the benefits of massage

Hippocrates: known as the father of medicine, believed all doctors needed to know how to use massage for healing purposes. Hippocrates called it anatripsis — 'the art of rubbing a part upward, not downward'

Holistic massage: a form of Swedish massage which takes into account not only the whole body including the mind and spirit

Homeopathy: treats like with like to build up the patient's resistance and immunity

Hypertonic drinks: a highly concentrated drink containing more sugar particles and electrolytes than the body's own fluids resulting in slower absorption than water

Glossary continued

Hypotonic drinks: weak solution containing fewer particles of sugar and electrolytes than the body's own fluids resulting in faster absorption into the body than water

Indian Head Massage: uses and adapts classic Swedish massage techniques for treating the scalp, face, neck, shoulders and upper arms

Insertion of muscle: the moving end of a muscle; the muscle always works by moving away from its insertion, towards the origin

Integral biology: the study of our environment's effect on our physical and mental health

Iridology: physical and psychological problems seen in changes in the iris of the eye

Isotonic drinks: approximately the same number of particles in water as body fluids resulting in absorption into the body as quickly, if not quicker than water

Kinesiology: testing of the muscles and energy meridians to discover and treat the body's imbalances

Lactic acid: by-product of oxygen deficiency in muscles; if muscle is tired and running out of oxygen but continues to be used (e.g. when an athlete over-exercises) then lactic acid builds up causing a burning pain and stiffness. The muscle needs to rest in order to allow a fresh supply of oxygen to reach it and the lactic acid to be removed.

Ling, Per Henrik (1776-1839): a physiologist and fencing master. He was from Sweden and massage is still referred to as Swedish massage because of his influence. In the eighteenth and nineteenth centuries he developed a system of movements which he found helpful for improving his health and maintaining his physical condition. These movements are known as the Ling System.

Local: refers to a particular area or effect as opposed to whole body

Lymphatic drainage massage: is a system of techniques that help the lymphatic system function effectively

Massage: use of hands or mechanical means to manipulate soft tissues of body

Medium: substance used to aid massage movements. Talc, oil, gel, cream and anti-inflammatory rubs can be used.

Muscle Energy technique (MET): a variety of techniques that involve restricted or resistive movements to stretch muscles

Muscle tone: the degree of contraction of muscle fibres; at any one time there are always some muscle fibres contracting and this gives the body its normal shape and posture

Neuromuscular technique (NMT): a form of friction movement holding thumb or finger over a sore point and increasing pressure gradually to the limit of the client's pain threshold

Oedema: swelling of tissue through increase of its interstitial fluid volume

Origin of muscle: the fixed end of a muscle; the muscle always works towards its origin

Osteopathy: manipulating the joints and bones to correct structural problems which will improve the body's functions

Palpation: feeling muscles to assess damage and how to treat it

Passive movement: movement which requires no client involvement

Percussion: stimulating stroke using repetitive, brisk movements which 'wake up', tone and energise the body

Petrissage: compression stroke used to manipulate tissues and muscles. Resembles kneading; helps to break down tension.

Physiotherapy: the use of physical exercises, massage and the application of pressure to relieve physical pain and muscular tension

Pressure points: points along the energy meridians

Pressure techniques: those that require application of pressure, usually from palm or heel of hand, fist, fingers or thumbs

Proteins: necessary for the growth and formation of new tissues, and also for repairing damaged tissues

Record card: an information sheet with all the client's personal details on and the treatments given

Referral area: area associated with another area of the body used in treatment when one area cannot be touched; e.g. if knee is damaged the knee's referral area, the elbow, can be treated instead

Reflexology: specialised foot massage treating the whole person by using the feet as 'maps' of the body. There are points or zones that correspond to organs and systems of the body. By pressing on one of these points, the corresponding organ in the body is affected

Reiki/spiritual healing: the use of the healer's hands on different parts of the body to draw energy to the patient's body promoting healing, balance and relaxation

Shiatsu: system of applying pressure to certain points on the body to improve circulation and health. It is performed with the client clothed.

Glossary continued

Soft Tissue Release (STR): combination of pressure and movement causing the muscle fibres to lengthen and stretch

Stress: is any factor that threatens our physical or mental well-being. There are two types of stress: positive, which can help some people perform to the best of their abilities, and negative, which is any factor causing us to respond by worrying, panicking or losing our concentration.

Superficial: surface of body; area closest to skin

Swedish massage: system of massage movements developed by and named after Swedish physiologist Per Henrik Ling. Movements were called effleurage, petrissage and percussion.

Tabla: superficial tapping movement using the tops of the fingers or the heels of the hands

Toxin: substance that can harm or damage the body if not removed; may be ingested or a by-product of body's functioning

Tsubo: Japanese name for the points of the body used in massage (based on Ancient Chinese practice)

Vibration: manual or mechanical method of moving flesh with gentle vibrations; can be stimulating or relaxing.

Waste: substances produced by body's functions which need to be removed in order for body to continue working effectively, e.g. carbon dioxide, urea

Working position: stance used by therapist to carry out treatment

Yoga: teaches the learner to have control over the mind and body through physical exercise.

Index

A

acne rosacea	13
acne vulgaris	13
acupressure	226, 229, 232
acupuncture	226, 229, 230, 232
aerobic system	206, 207
aftercare advice	99, 155, 232
Alexander technique	227, 232
almond oil	67, 181, 182, 210, 225
alopecia	182
anaemia	15, 18
anaerobic system	206, 207
analgesic effect	145
aniseed	225
arnica	225
Aromatherapy	10, 224-6
arteriosclerosis	16
arthritis	93, 117, 182
atherosclerosis	16
atony	19
atrophy	19
aura	142, 147-8, 151, 154, 161, 170
Ayurvedic medicine	9, 178, 227, 232

B

Bach flower remedies	227, 230, 232
basalt stone	144-5, 151, 153-4, 159
beating	35, 36
Bell's palsy	26, 93, 117, 182
bitter almond	225
bitter fennel	225
blood pressure	16, 74, 77, 107, 109, 178, 208, 210, 232
body language	89, 91
body work	227
boils	13
Bowen technique	227, 232

C

camphor	225
cancer	14, 16, 18, 93, 117
carbohydrate (energy) drinks	212
carbohydrates	208, 209, 211, 232
cardiovascular system	37, 207, 208
care (of the therapist)	101-103
carrier oil	224-6, 232
cassia	225
cell	75, passim
chakra	146-8
champissage	180
chiropractic	227, 232
cholesterol	16, 210
cinnamon bark	225
circulatory system	15, 77, 119, 178
client modesty	97
closed questions	85, 90, 91
coconut oil	181, 182
colour therapy	227, 230
communication	89-91
compresses	201
compression	195, 197, 198, 199
confidentiality	92
consent	93
cramp	19, 197, 202, 211
creatine phosphate	206
cross-fibre friction	33, 34, 195, 199
crystal therapy	148, 227
cupping	36

D

dandruff	182
data protection	92
deep friction	195
dehydration	149, 211
dermatitis	13, 132

Index continued

desquamation   75, 233
diet   208
digestive system   79
dwarf pine   225

E

ear candling   228
eczema   13, 182
effleurage   30-32, *passim*
elecampane   225
electro magnetic field   142
emulsion   40
endorphins   110
essential oils   224-6

F

fats   209-210
fibrositis   19
fluid replacement drink   211
fluid retention   117, 120, 145, 153, 195
fluids   208-212
folliculitis   13
friction   33-34, 133, 150, 180, *passim*
fungal conditions   14, 85

H

hacking   35-36
haemophilia   16, 93
haemorrhoids   16
healing crisis   99, 155, 184
heart   15, 16, 93, 119
hepatitis A, B, C   16
herbalism   228
herpes   14
high blood pressure   16
Hodgkin's lymphoma   18
holistic approach   106
homecare   133
homeopathy   228

homeostasis   107, 120
horseradish   225
hygiene   82, 84-89, 155
hypertonic drink   211
hypnotherapy   228
hypotonic drink   211
hyssop   225

I

immune system   110, 120, 195, 210
impetigo   14, 86
inflammation   94, 145, 149, 178, 201
integral biology   92, 106
integumentary system   12
iridology   228
isotonic drin   211

K

kinesiology   228
Kneipp theory   143

L

leukaemia   16, 131
Ling, Per Henrik   10, 30
low blood pressure   16
lymphatic system   17, 18, 78, 119

M

marble   144-5, 154-6
massage
   case studies   64-71, 122-7, 136-9,
                              157-169, 185-9, 213-221
   contraindications to   93-94, 117, 131
   equipment for   96-97, 154, 183
   in a care setting   100
   mediums   40, 145
   psychological benefits of 74, 146, 225
   reactions to   14, 41, 99, 155, 184
   routine   42-63
   working positions   103

massage types
  classical/Swedish   29-39, *passim*
  connective tissue (CTM)   196
  corrective   199
  Indian head   177-184, 190-2
  infant (and child)   129-135
  lymphatic drainage   115-121
  on-site   111-113
  preventative   198-9
  scalp   181
  sports   193-9
  stone therapy   141-6, 148-156
  Thai   230

maximum effort   206-207
meditation   104, 227, 230
Mohs scale   144
motor neurone disease   26, 93
multiple sclerosis   27
muscle energy technique   196
muscular system   19, 76, 119, 178
mustard   225
mustard oil   181, 182
myalgic encephalomyelitis (ME)   27
myositis   25

N
naturopathy   228
nervous system   26, 78, 93, 110, 120, 131, 207
neuralgia   27
neuritis   27
neurolinguistic programming   228
neuromuscular technique   196

O
oedema   78, 93, 201, 235
olive oil   181, 182
origanum   225

osteopathy   229
osteoporosis   93, 117, 131, 183

P
palpation   200
Parkinson's disease   26, 93
passive movements   38
patch test   41
pennyroyal   225
percussion   35-37, *passim*
petrissage   32-33, 133, 150, 179, 194
phlebitis   16, 93
physiotherapy   10, 229
piezoelectric effect   151
posture   101-102
pounding   36
pregnancy   93, 94, 117, 226
pressure points   9, 181
pressured stroking   153
protein   205, 209
psoriasis   13

R
record card   65-66, 92
referral procedure   93-94, 131
reflexology   229, 230
reiki   229, 230
respiratory system   80
rheumatism   94, 117
rubbing   9, 32, 33, 180
rue   225
rupture   25, 203

S
sage   225
salt tablets   211
sassafras   225
savin   225
savory   225

Index continued

sciatica	26, 93
sensitive skin	41
sesame oil	181, 182
Shiatsu	229
skeletal system	79, 178
skin	12-14, 40-41
soft tissue release	194, 196
southernwood	225
spasm	8, 25, 100
spasticity	25
sports drinks	211
sprain	25, 131, 203
strain	25, 79, 204
stress	16, 25, 26, 107-110
stretching	196, 197

T

tabla	180
tansy	225
tapotement	37, 148, 150
thrombosis	16, 93
thuja	225
tinea corporis	14
tinea pedis	14, 85
trigger point	152

U

urinary system	80, 149

V

varicose veins	17, 94
vasoconstriction	145
verrucas	14
vibration	38, 151, 199
viral conditions	14

W

warts	14
water	99, 106, 143, 149, 201, 210-211
wintergreen	225
wormseed	225
wormwood	225

Y

yoga	104, 230